Introduction to Psychology of Mental Health

By Joy Bose and Siva Prasad Bose

Contents

Dedication

<hr>

This book is dedicated to all those who are suffering from mental health related issues and stress in India.

Preface

In this book, we study some of the techniques on how to improve our mental health and how it is composed of different factors.

We first discuss what is mental health, which is the absence of mental disorders. Then we discuss a few different types of mental disorders such as schizophrenia and depression, showing the biological, social and psychological factors behind each of the disorders. Then we discuss in detail stress, which is a common mental disorder that affects our well-being. We discuss theories of stress and how to combat stress using techniques such as logotherapy, CBT and positive psychology.

It is hoped that reading these factors and techniques will enable the reader of how psychology can be applied to enhance one's mental health in daily life.

Important Note

This Book is intended to be a guide for people suffering from stress and other mental health issues and only serves as an initial guide. As a person affected, it is advisable to additionally seek professional advice or to consult a doctor / psychologist / psychiatrist.

About the authors

Joy Bose is a data scientist by profession and also a part-time community well-being volunteer with National Institute of Mental Health and Neurosciences (NIMHANS) in Bangalore, India. He has more than 5 years of experience in giving well-being seminars and counseling men for men's community centers in Bangalore and New Delhi, India, affiliated with a Non-Governmental Organization called Save Indian Family Foundation. He has a diploma in creative hypnotherapy from Northern College of Creative Hypnotherapy, UK, has practiced mindfulness meditation for a number of years, received training as a well-being volunteer with NIMHANS, Bangalore, India and has completed a part time online master's degree in psychology of Mental Health from King's College, London, UK. His other education consists of a PhD in Computer Science from University of Manchester, UK and a B. Eng degree in Computer Science from National Institute of Technology, Allahabad, India.

Siva Prasad Bose is a retired electrical engineer and writer of introductory guides on aspects of law in India.

Acknowledgement for writing this book

This book incorporates teachings in stress management and suicide prevention learnt from previous trainings at NIMHANS and NCOCH, learnings from the masters course in psychology and neuroscience of mental health in King's College, courses on positive psychology from Coursera, and experience out of counselling of various people and seminars related to well-being given for the Save Indian Family Foundation NGO.

In preparing this book, the authors would like to acknowledge advice from different sources including Dr. Arvind Raj from NIMHANS, the men's community center in Bangalore, Jonathan and Ray from NCOCH (Northern College of Creative Hypnotherapy), UK and countless discussions with various people. Special thanks to Vijay Sahu who gave a number of mental health workshops and is also a trained well-being volunteer from NIMHANS.

Chapter 1: What is Mental Health

In this chapter, we introduce the concept of mental health and give some examples of mental disorders.

1.1 Definition of mental health

Mental health is overall well-being that is a combination of emotional, psychological, social and other kinds of well-being. It can be said to be an absence of mental disorders. It also encompasses many angles such as enjoyment of life, freedom to live as one wants to, psychological resilience, and self-actualization.

According to World Health Organization (WHO), mental health is a state of well-being in which the individual realizes his or her abilities, can cope with the normal stresses of life, can work productively and fruitfully, and can contribute to his or her community.

Mental health has a biological, a psychological and a social basis. In combination, we can say it is a bio-psycho-social phenomenon.

From one viewpoint, mental health means the freedom from impairment resulting from mental disorders. As per the 1983 mental health act in UK, a mental disorder may be understood as a disorder or disability of the mind.

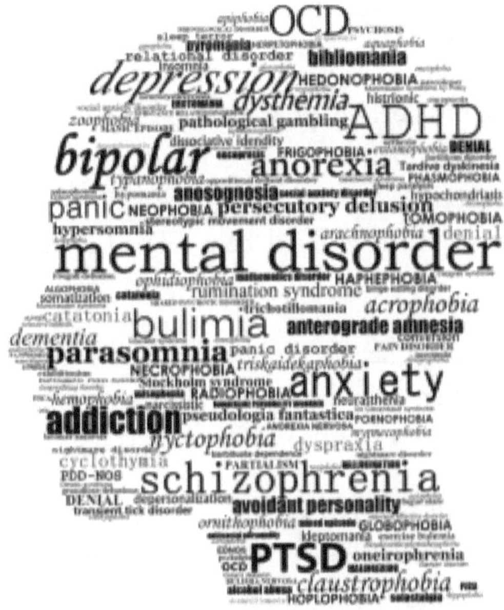

Figure: A picture showing the variety of mental health illnesses. Paget Michael Creelman, CC BY-SA 4.0 <https://creativecommons.org/licenses/by-sa/4.0>, via Wikimedia Commons

1.2 Examples of mental disorders

Examples of mental disorders include the following:

- affective disorders, such as depression and bipolar disorder.
- schizophrenia and delusional disorders; neurotic disorders; organic mental disorders, such as dementia and delirium.
- personality and behavioral changes caused by brain injury; importantly from a legal perspective, personality disorders.
- mental and behavioral disorders caused by psychoactive substance use.
- eating disorders.
- learning disabilities; autistic spectrum disorders; and behavioral and emotional disorders of children and young people.

1.3 Why mental health

Mental health is a very important and often overlooked issue in the fast-paced world today. Unlike physical health issues, where people rush to seek treatment from a qualified doctor or medical practitioner, there is still a kind of stigma over mental health in some cultures, due to which some people are reluctant to seek professional help related to mental health.

The scale of stress and other mental health problems can be illustrated by taking the example of IT workers in India. Following are the findings from a few surveys of IT workers:

- A 2022 survey of Indian IT workers found the following: 34% Indian IT professionals feel frequently stressed at work and heavy workload is the top stressor at work for 51% of the survey respondents.
- In a survey of 1000 corporate employees by Holmes and Rahe, around 56% of the respondents had musculoskeletal symptoms. 22% had newly diagnosed hypertension, 10% had diabetes, 36% had dyslipidemia, 54% had depression, anxiety and insomnia, 40% had obesity.
- In a Covid time survey, 80% of Indian IT professionals experienced deadline pressures, long working hours, regular multi-tasking, and difficulty in maintaining work–life balance.
- A 2023 survey by ADP research institute found that about 76% Indian workers felt stress had a negative impact on work performance.

In spite of the scale of the problem, there is a lack of mental health support. Some IT companies in India offer 3rd party counselling services, also called Employee Assistance Programs or EAPs, to their employees, including phone support and online support in case of stress and other mental health issues. Examples of such EAP services include Optum, 1to1Help and others.

However, these are not always effective: employees may worry the information might be shared with the employer and negatively affect them. The Indian government does not give much support either. Support from mental health NGOs is limited.

IT workers in India are stressed due to various reasons like high workload, family issues, financial problems like EMIs of housing loans, uncertainty of work etc. The support given by IT companies and government is insufficient. Therefore, there exists a gap in the provision of mental health services to Indian IT workers.

References:

- https://spacelift.io/blog/are-it-jobs-stressful
- https://www.ncbi.nlm.nih.gov/pmc/articles/PMC4439723/
- https://www.ncbi.nlm.nih.gov/pmc/articles/PMC11006029/
- https://economictimes.indiatimes.com/jobs/hr-policies-trends/76-of-indian-workers-say-stress-negatively-impacting-work-shows-survey/articleshow/102810905.cms?from=mdr

1.4 Conclusion

In this chapter, we have briefly gone over the definition of mental health and discussed some types of mental disorders. We also discussed the need for mental health support, taking Indian IT employees as an example.

Chapter 2: Positive psychology for mental health and well-being

In this chapter, we discuss a few techniques derived from positive psychology, that can be used to cultivate happiness and a positive outlook, that leads to overall mental well-being.

2.1 Introduction to Positive Psychology

Positive psychology was first popularized by Martin Seligman in 1998. It refers to scientifically researched methods to increase happiness and well-being in our lives, leading to an improved quality of life.

Positive psychology for mental health includes paying more attention to building on positive behaviors and traits already present in individuals. Positive psychology interventions aim to boost positive emotions and help clients find meaning in life.

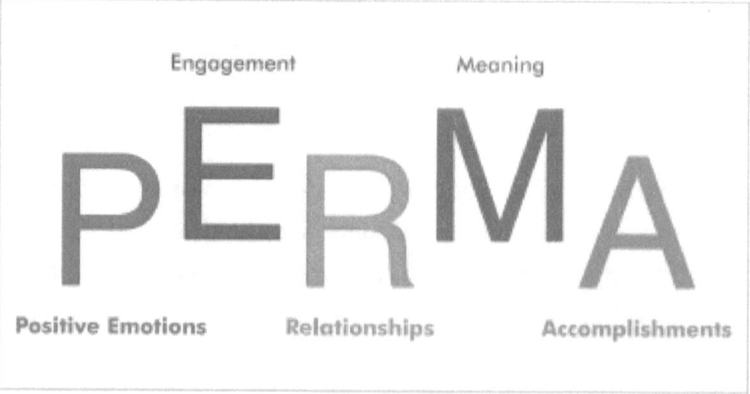

Figure: PERMA model. Rulebased, CC BY-SA 4.0 <https://creativecommons.org/licenses/by-sa/4.0>, via Wikimedia Commons

One of the models used in positive psychology is called the **PERMA model**. It consists of the following components:

- **Positive Emotions**: These include cultivating emotions such as happiness, satisfaction, pride, joy etc.
- **Engagement**: This includes indulging in activities and hobbies which we enjoy and are genuinely interested in, and which bring us into a state of flow.
- **Relationships**: This involves cultivating meaningful relationships with other people.
- **Meaning**: This involves having a sense of purpose and finding out the "why".
- **Accomplishments**: These include the pursuit of success and mastery in our activities.

Cultivated together, these components can lead to a sense of well-being. We should consciously try and cultivate each of these.

2.2 Five steps to mental wellbeing

The five steps to mental wellbeing is taken from the UK NHS toolkit of the same name 'Five steps to mental wellbeing.'

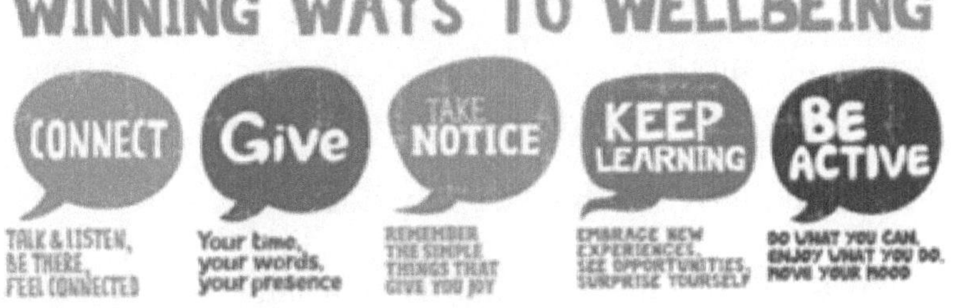

Figure: NHS UK. Winning Ways to Wellbeing

The five steps are as follows:

- 'connect' — connect with the people around you;
- 'give to others' — such as volunteering at your local centre, can improve your mental wellbeing and help you build new social networks;
- 'be mindful / take notice' — be more aware of the present moment, including your thoughts and feelings, your body, and the world around you.
- 'keep learning' — learning new skills can give you a sense of achievement and new confidence, so why not sign up for that cooking course, start learning to play a musical instrument
- 'be active' — you don't have to go to the gym, which I'm pleased about — take a walk, go cycling, or play a game of football

Reference: https://www.nhs.uk/mental-health/self-help/guides-tools-and-activities/five-steps-to-mental-wellbeing/

2.3 Happiness hormones and stress hormones

A lot of the communication in our brain happens due to chemicals called neurotransmitters or different types of hormones. These chemicals govern our different emotions and response to different types of situations. As long as these chemicals remain in balance, we can have a healthy outlook and deal with adversities. But when they go out of balance, that is when we can get into all kinds of mental problems.

A few of the happiness related hormones are listed as follows:

- **Serotonin**: This neurotransmitter contributes significantly to feelings of well-being and happiness. Levels can be boosted by engaging in acts of kindness, such as helping others or volunteering, as well as through exercise, sunlight exposure, and positive social interactions.

- **Oxytocin**: This hormone is triggered on the sensation of touch from our loved ones, such as a hug, and is also associated with happiness.
- **Dopamine**: This is another of the happiness hormones, and is associated with the feeling of reward or accomplishment, and is released when someone praises us, or we accomplish something.
- **Endorphins**: These hormones are released when we exercise our body e.g. by running or doing yoga, and also are triggered when we meditate or when we laugh. Endorphins are the most common type of happiness hormone.

There are also a few stress related hormones, which are markers of stress in our body. Some of them are as follows:

- **Cortisol**: This is the main stress hormone. It makes us more alert and ready to face the perceived threat or threats, in the short term. In the long term, when we are subjected to a prolonged period of stress, this can have an adverse effect on our health.
- **Adrenaline**: This is the hormone that gives some people a high, and is triggered by the fight or flight response such as a simulated danger in a roller coaster. This too is harmful in the long term.

Knowing about these hormones, the best way to increase our happiness would be to do activities that trigger the happiness hormones as often as we can. For example, this can be done by having regular exercises or yoga, helping people around us in different ways, and doing meditation.

2.4 Cultivating mental well-being by paying attention to simple pleasures in life

Sometimes, simple pleasures in life such as having a good time chatting with friends in a cosy and relaxing environment with good food and drink can bring us happiness. We can regularly schedule such meetings with close friend, and it will be something for us to look forward to. This is the essence of the Danish idea of **Hygge**, and in some ways also similar to the Swedish idea of **Fika**.

In our life, we should knowingly try and make time for such simple pleasures regularly or once every few weeks.

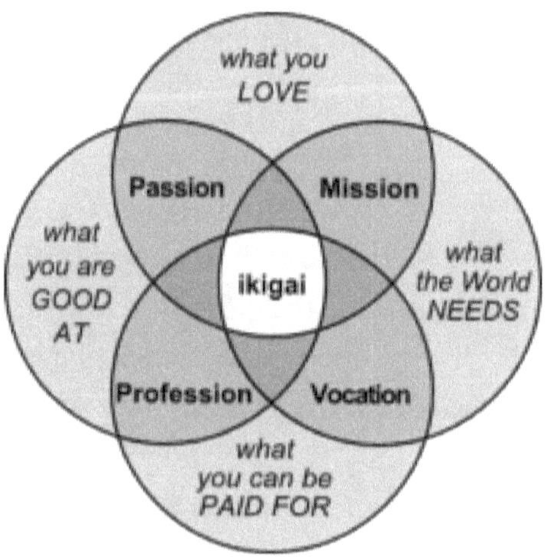

Figure: Illustration of Ikigai

2.5 Cultivating mental well-being by discovering our ikigai

Ikigai is a Japanese term meaning life's purpose or calling. The Venn diagram about Ikigai in the figure above gives some idea of what Ikigai means. In short, it is the intersection of what we love to do, what we are good at, what the world needs, and what the world is willing to pay us.

Sometimes, we get trapped into careers and jobs that pay well but which we do not like, or things that we like but do not pay well, or things that we want but we are not so good at. It is worth to spend some time to figure out which kind of career can fulfill our ikigai.

Ideally, we should be able to find purpose and meaning in whatever we do. However, in the long term we should aim to cultivate a career which matches our ikigai, since that is the way to maximize our happiness with our work.

2.6 Conclusion

In this chapter, we have briefly discussed about positive psychology and how it can be applied in the area of mental health. By consciously cultivating strategies for happiness and mental well-being such as those taken from positive psychology, we can focus on the more positive aspects of life rather than being bogged down by the negativity of the stressful situations.

Chapter 3: Example of a mental disorder: Depression

In the previous chapters, we discussed some basics about mental health and how positive psychology can be used to improve one's mental health. In this chapter, we look at depression, which is a common and important mental health disorder.

3.1 What is depression

As per DSM-5, depression is diagnosed if 5 or more of the following symptoms are diagnosed in the same 2-week period and out of these, at least one of the symptoms includes depressed mood or loss of interest or pleasure:

- depressed mood
- diminished interest or pleasure
- insomnia
- psychomotor retardation
- daily fatigue or loss of energy
- feelings of worthlessness
- diminished ability to think or concentrate
- recurrent thoughts of death
- impairment of social or occupational functioning

Depression affects about one in five adults, median onset is about 25 years of age, leading cause of morbidity (DALYs — disability adjusted life year)

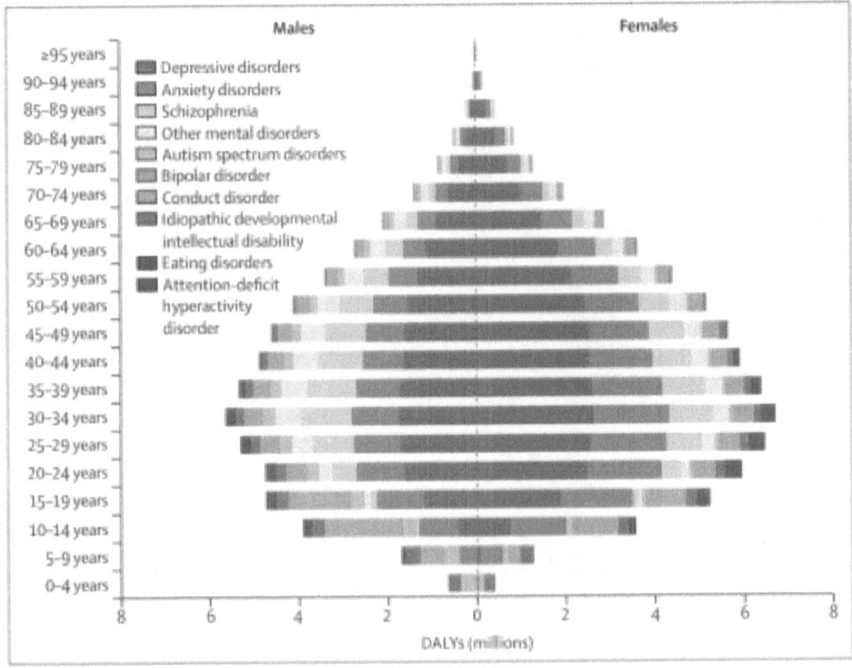

Figure: DALYs (disability adjusted life years) lost due to depression and other mental health disorders. Taken from global burden of disease study 2019

3.2 Biological, genetic, and environmental causes of depression

The cause of depression is said to be one third genetic, and two third environmental (social traumas, financial, health problems).

Depression is said to be associated with the change in inflammatory markers in immune system.

There is a monoamine hypothesis of depression, which postulates that depression is due to deficiency of neurotransmitter levels in the brain.

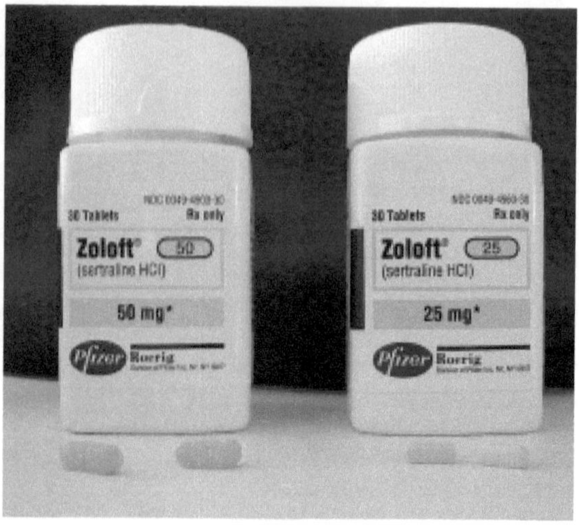

Figure: Sertraline (Zoloft) is an antidepressant, used primarily to treat major depression in adults. Ragesoss, Public domain, via Wikimedia Commons

3.3 Treatment for depression

A common treatment for depression is using antidepressants. These are pharmacological pills, usually prescribed by a psychiatrist after proper diagnosis, that can help to reduce the symptoms of depression: and lead to an increased number of new neurons.

Another common treatment is using CBT, which we will discuss in the following subsection.

3.4 Cognitive behavioral therapy (CBT) for depression

CBT is based on the cognitive model, that postulates that negative thoughts and views about oneself, the world and future, affect one's behavior. CBT is one of the popular talking therapies available today, since it has good research proving its effectiveness, is relatively quick and has few or no side effects as compared to other options.

CBT treatment for depression includes the following:

- **Identifying negative thoughts, emotions and behaviors**: The client is encouraged to monitor their automatic thoughts, emotions and behaviors that occur every day. This can be done by the clients reflecting and writing down their thoughts in different situations or at different times of the day, especially when they are feeling depressed. The help of structured questionnaires, worksheets and forms can be taken for the same. The client is enabled to make a connection between the negative thoughts and depression.

- **Challenging negative thought patterns**: Once the negative thoughts are identified, the client is encouraged to examine each thought and challenge the assumptions underlying such thoughts and emotions, sometimes with evidence of the opposite. For example, if the thought is "I am a failure", the client is encouraged to bring to mind instances in their life where they have been successful and not a failure. For example, they might be handling their finances quite well or taking care of their family. This can also be done for events that occurred in the client's life during the day or the week. The client is enabled to reframe the automatic negative thoughts into more realistic appraisals about the situation or event.

- **Action plans and activities to strengthen positive behaviors**: The client is encouraged to cultivate positive emotions and experiences. This can be done by encouraging them to bring to mind positive memories and positive incidents during the day. This enables them to focus more on the positive incidents rather than only the negative ones. Action plans can be formulated, consisting of small activities throughout the day that cause the clients to have a sense of accomplishment and achievement, thus encouraging positive thoughts.

- **Inculcating skills for problem solving and stress

management: The CBT therapist encourages the client to inculcate skills to deal with problems and stress in a better way. Some practices for stress management can include deep breathing and mindfulness meditation.

3.5 Conclusion

In this chapter we have discussed depression, which is one of the important mental health disorders.

Chapter 4: Example of a mental disorder: Schizophrenia

In this chapter, we discuss schizophrenia, which is a type of psychosis, in which a person has difficulty in distinguishing what is real from what is not. We focus on its bio-psycho-social model to understand the factors that lead to a diagnosis of schizophrenia.

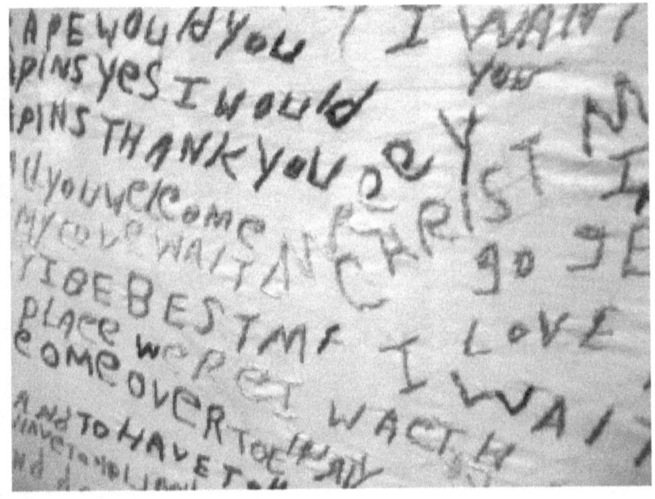

Figure: Cloth embroidered by a schizophrenic patient, now showcased at the Glore Psychiatric Museum. cometstarmoon, CC BY 2.0 <https://creativecommons.org/licenses/by/2.0>, via Wikimedia Commons

4.1 What is schizophrenia

Schizophrenia is a mental disorder characterized by two or more of the following symptoms during a one-month period as per DSM-5 (American Psychiatric Association, 2013):

Two or more symptoms among the following:

- hallucinations
- delusions
- disorganized speech
- disorganized or catatonic behavior,
- negative symptoms,
- and which are not attributable to any other condition.

It is a form of psychosis.

Schizophrenia has the following experiences in the subjects:

- Hears voices: cannot filter our irrelevant stimuli
- Feels others can read their mind
- Subject gets paranoid: cuts off social interaction
- Often occurs in more creative people (see the film, a beautiful mind, which beautifully illustrates the schizophrenia of John Nash, a brilliant mathematician who also won a Nobel prize)
- Some people can have multiple episodes at various intervals

As per the ICD-10 definition (World Health Organization, 1983), psychosis can be diagnosed if the subject reports the presence of auditory hallucinations, delusions and abnormalities of behavior such as catatonia, overexcitement and retardation, within a short period of time.

Schizophrenia was first identified by the German psychologist Emil Kraepelin in the 19th century as 'dementia praecox', an incurable and progressively deteriorating disease. It affects a significant percentage of the population, across different countries, and results in a significant cost to both affected individuals as well as the wider society, including mental health costs, a reduced Quality of Life (Narvaez et al., 2008) and the number of Quality Adjusted Life Years or QALYs lost (Carr et al., 2006).

Figure: The brain of a schizophrenic. BruceBlaus, CC BY-SA 4.0 <https://creativecommons.org/licenses/by-sa/4.0>, via Wikimedia Commons

4.2 Biology of schizophrenia

Schizophrenia is associated with increased dopamine (neurotransmitter) synthesis.

There is an important hypothesis called the Dopamine hypothesis of schizophrenia, which attempts to explain the cause of schizophrenia. It states that dopamine neurotransmitters disturbances in the mesolimbic pathway and prefrontal cortex of the brain could be a cause of the positive symptoms of schizophrenia, such as seeing and hearing hallucinations.

Similarly, the negative and cognitive symptoms of schizophrenia, such as diminished cognitive ability, are associated with the meso-cortical pathway of the brain.

In schizophrenics, we can commonly observe a decrease of grey matter in the brain: loss of brain tissue. This is also responsible for cognitive difficulties in the person.

4.3 Environmental and developmental factors of schizophrenia

Schizophrenia is associated with environmental factors and triggers such as stress.

Social anxiety and depression in childhood may be linked to schizophrenia in later years.

Being abused as a child can increase one's risk of psychosis and schizophrenia.

Social fragmentation in big cities, and being a member of migrant or minority ethnic groups is associated with a higher risk of schizophrenia.

4.4 Genetic factors of schizophrenia

Ripke et al. (2014) identified 108 independently associated genetic loci that function as markers of schizophrenia. So if a person's genes contain these loci, that means that the person has a higher risk of becoming schizophrenic. However, since there are other factors such as environmental factors at play, it is not necessary that every person who has such genes will end up becoming schizophrenic.

Reference: Schizophrenia Working Group of the Psychiatric Genomics Consortium. Biological insights from 108 schizophrenia-associated genetic loci. Nature. 2014 Jul 24;511(7510):421-7. doi: 10.1038/nature13595. Epub 2014 Jul 22. PMID: 25056061; PMCID: PMC4112379.

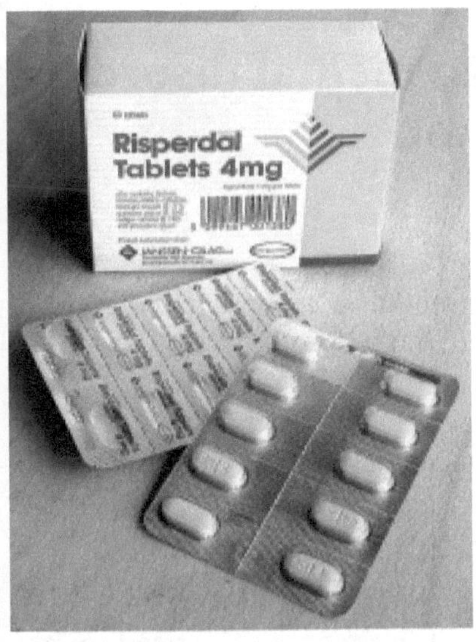

Figure: Risperidone (trade name Risperdal) is a common atypical antipsychotic medication. Housed, CC BY-SA 3.0 <https://creativecommons.org/licenses/by-sa/3.0>, via Wikimedia Commons

4.5 Treatment of schizophrenia

Schizophrenia is often treated by antipsychotic drugs. These drugs block the dopamine receptors in the brain of the person, which can be said to be associated with the positive symptoms of schizophrenia such as hallucinations, as per the dopamine hypothesis.

4.6 Conclusion

In this chapter, we have discussed schizophrenia which is a mental disorder that causes hallucinations and other symptoms in a person. We have briefly discussed the bio, psycho and social factors that are responsible for this disorder.

Chapter 5: Example of a mental disorder: Addiction

In this chapter, we discuss a common mental disorder which is addiction.

5.1 Introduction to addiction

In addiction, the use of a drug of abuse is increased to maintain euphoria or avoid dysphoria or withdrawal.

Examples of addiction include: addiction to drugs, alcohol, even addiction to mobile phones. The addicted subject feels the need to take more and more of the drugs to get the same pleasurable sensations and avoid the withdrawal symptoms.

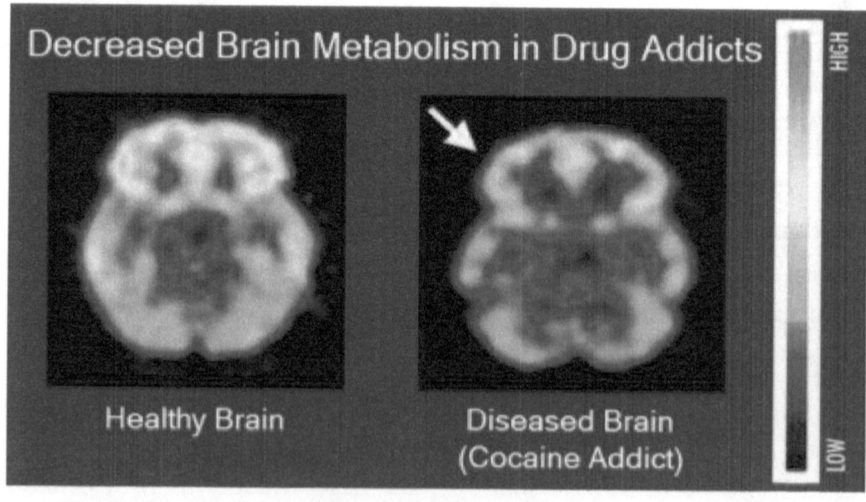

Figure: Healthy brain vs brain of a cocaine addict. Drs. Nora Volkow and Heinrich Schelbert, National Institutes of Health (NIH), Public domain, via Wikimedia Commons

5.2 Biology of addiction

In the addicted subject's brain, the number of receptors increases, the number of neurotransmitters decreases, reinforcing properties of the drug gradually decrease (tolerance), and the body's dependence on the drug increases. The subject has to take more of the drug to get the same pleasure.

The biological factors associated with addiction are as follows: In addicted subjects, the reward pathway of the brain (related to modulation of the dopamine system) is hijacked by addictive drugs. For example, nicotine and MDMA are associated with increase in the firing of dopamine neurons in the nucleus accumbens area of the brain, that is associated with pleasure.

5.3 Genetic factors related to addiction

There are multiple twin studies (studies on twins, at least one of whom is suffering from addiction) and adoption studies (studies on genetic twins who were adopted into different families) which suggest that the transmission of alcoholism or addiction to alcohol is determined more by genetics than the environment.

5.4 Social and developmental factors of addiction

Social and developmental factors of addiction include the following: economic deprivation, drug use among peers, neighborhood disorganization, family conflict and behavior problems in childhood. These increase the risk of addiction for those who are genetically already susceptible.

5.5 Conclusion

In this chapter, we have discussed the mental disorder of addiction and briefly gone through some of the biological and social factors that can make a person more at risk of addiction.

Chapter 6: Example of a Mental Health Disorder: Dementia and Alzheimer's Disease

In this chapter, we explore dementia, with a particular focus on Alzheimer's disease, which is the most common form of dementia. We will examine its characteristics, causes, and potential management strategies, using a bio-psycho-social framework to understand this progressive mental disorder that significantly impacts memory and cognition.

6.1 What is Dementia and Alzheimer's

Dementia is an umbrella term for a range of progressive neurological disorders characterized by a decline in cognitive functioning, including memory, reasoning, and communication skills, severe enough to interfere with daily life.

According to the Diagnostic and Statistical Manual of Mental Disorders (DSM-5), dementia, now classified under "Major Neurocognitive Disorder," involves significant cognitive decline in one or more domains—such as memory, attention, or problem-solving—beyond what is expected from normal aging, accompanied by a loss of independence in everyday activities.

Alzheimer's disease accounts for 60-80% of dementia cases. It is a specific neurodegenerative condition marked by the gradual loss of memory and cognitive abilities. Symptoms of Alzheimer's typically include:

- Memory loss, particularly of recent events
- Difficulty in planning or solving problems

- Confusion with time or place
- Challenges in understanding visual images or spatial relationships
- Problems with language, such as forgetting words
- Misplacing items and inability to retrace steps
- Withdrawal from social activities
- Changes in mood or personality, such as increased irritability or apathy

Alzheimer's often begins subtly, with mild memory lapses, and progresses to severe impairment, where individuals may no longer recognize loved ones or perform basic tasks. It typically affects older adults, with prevalence increasing significantly after age 65, though early-onset forms can occur before this age.

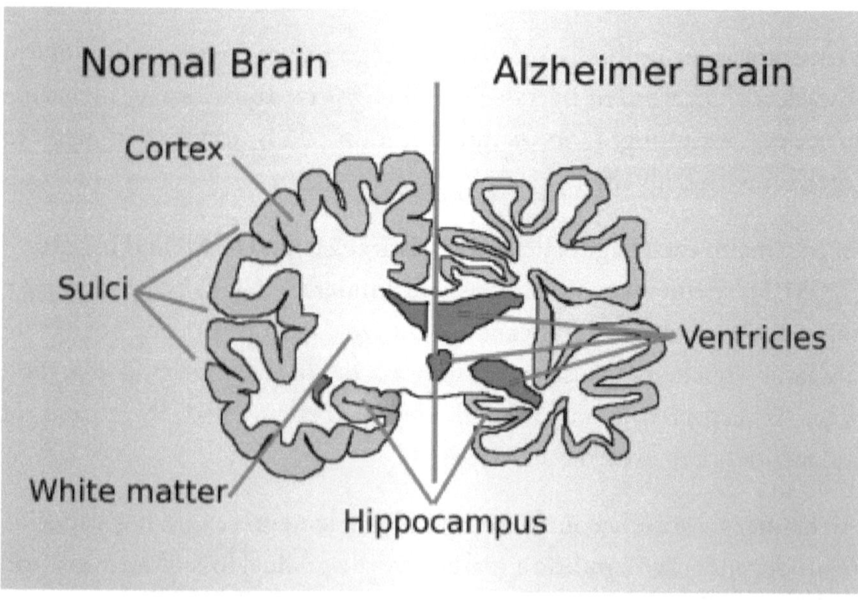

Figure: Drawing comparing how a brain of an Alzheimer disease patient is affected to a normal brain. Garrondo, Public domain, via Wikimedia Commons

6.2 Biology of Dementia and Alzheimer's

The biological basis of Alzheimer's involves structural and chemical changes in the brain. Two hallmark features are:

- Amyloid Plaques: These are abnormal clumps of beta-amyloid protein that accumulate between neurons, disrupting communication.
- Neurofibrillary Tangles: These are twisted strands of tau protein that build up inside neurons, impairing their ability to transport nutrients and eventually leading to cell death.

These changes lead to a loss of neurons and synapses, particularly in areas like the hippocampus (crucial for memory) and the cerebral cortex (involved in reasoning and language). Neurotransmitter imbalances, especially a reduction in acetylcholine—a chemical messenger vital for memory and learning—further exacerbate cognitive decline.

Other changes are:

- Brain Shrinkage: There is a progressive shrinkage of the brain, especially in areas involved with memory such as the hippocampus and frontal cortex.
- Neurotransmitter Changes: Patients with Alzheimer's typically show reduced levels of acetylcholine, a neurotransmitter important for memory and learning.

Research suggests inflammation and oxidative stress also play roles, as the brain struggles to clear damaged cells and debris. Over time, this neurodegeneration spreads, shrinking the brain's volume and impairing its functions.

6.3 Genetic Factors of Dementia and Alzheimer's

Certain genetic markers are associated with a higher risk of developing Alzheimer's:

- APOE-e4 gene increases the risk of late-onset Alzheimer's.
- Familial Alzheimer's (early-onset) may be caused by mutations in genes such as APP, PSEN1, and PSEN2. Twin studies suggest heritability of Alzheimer's is around 60-80%, but environmental triggers often determine whether genetic predisposition manifests as disease.

Reference: Gatz, M., et al. (2006). Role of genes and environments for explaining Alzheimer disease. Archives of General Psychiatry, 63(2), 168-174. DOI: 10.1001/archpsyc.63.2.168

6.4 Environmental and Developmental Factors of Dementia and Alzheimer's

While aging is the primary risk factor, environmental and lifestyle factors can influence the onset and progression of dementia and Alzheimer's. These include:

- Cardiovascular Health: Conditions like hypertension, diabetes, and high cholesterol increase risk by impairing blood flow to the brain.
- Head Trauma: Head injuries, such as those experienced by athletes or accident victims, are linked to higher dementia rates.
- Vascular disease: This is closely related to a type of dementia called vascular dementia. It is caused by reduced blood flow to the brain, often due to strokes or small vessel disease (micro-infarcts), which damage the brain tissue over time.
- Social Isolation: Lack of social engagement and intellectual stimulation may accelerate cognitive decline. This may be related to, for example, loneliness in older adults.
- Education and Cognitive Reserve: Lower educational

attainment is associated with higher risk, possibly due to less "cognitive reserve"—the brain's resilience built through mental activity.

- Chronic stress and poor sleep, common in fast-paced modern lifestyles, may also exacerbate risk by increasing inflammation and cortisol levels, which can damage brain cells over time.
- Other factors include lack of physical and cognitive ability, smoking and alcohol, and a poor diet with high sugar and low antioxidants.

6.5 Diagnosis and Assessment

Diagnosis is based on clinical evaluation, cognitive tests, and sometimes brain imaging (like MRI or PET scans) to observe shrinkage and protein accumulation.

Common screening tools include:

- Mini-Mental State Examination (MMSE)
- Montreal Cognitive Assessment (MoCA)

Often, family members are the first to notice signs of cognitive decline, and a full medical, psychiatric, and neuropsychological evaluation is recommended.

6.6 Treatment and Management of Dementia and Alzheimer's

Currently, there is no cure for Alzheimer's or most forms of dementia, but treatments can manage symptoms and improve quality of life. Common approaches include the following:

- Pharmacological Interventions: Cholinesterase inhibitors (e.g., donepezil, rivastigmine) boost acetylcholine levels, temporarily improving memory and cognition in mild to moderate Alzheimer's. Memantine, an NMDA receptor antagonist, helps regulate glutamate activity in moderate to severe cases. Antidepressants and antipsychotics may be used to treat behavioral symptoms.

- Cognitive Stimulation Therapy (CST): This involves structured activities—like puzzles, music, or reminiscence exercises—to engage memory and reasoning skills, slowing cognitive decline.
- Lifestyle Modifications: Regular physical exercise, a Mediterranean diet rich in antioxidants, and mental activities (e.g., reading, learning new skills) are shown to delay symptom progression by supporting brain health.
- Psychosocial Support: Counseling and support groups for patients and caregivers address emotional strain, fostering resilience and coping strategies.
- Emerging research explores anti-amyloid therapies and lifestyle interventions to prevent or delay onset, though these remain experimental.
- Other Non-Pharmacological Strategies include behavioural therapy for managing agitation or aggression through structured routines, mindfulness and reminiscence therapy for helping patients remain calm and feel secure. A daily routine and structure leading to a familiar environment reduces confusion and anxiety in patients.

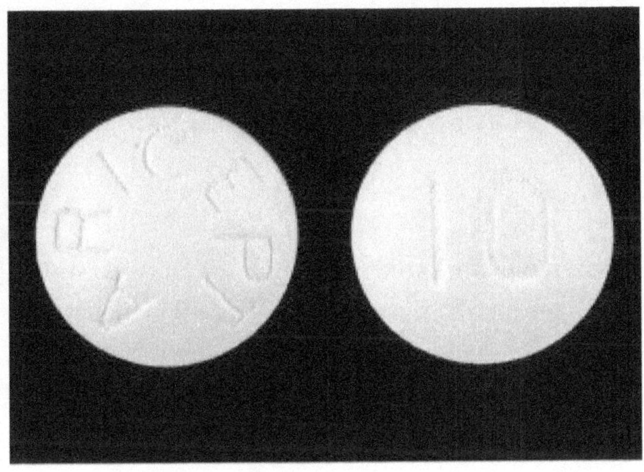

Figure: A 10 mg pill of Donepezil (Aricept), a cholinesterase inhibitor commonly prescribed for Alzheimer's. NLM, Public domain, via Wikimedia Commons.

6.7 Conclusion

In this chapter, we have examined dementia, focusing on Alzheimer's disease as a prevalent and impactful mental disorder. We explored its biological underpinnings—plaques, tangles, and neurotransmitter loss—alongside environmental and genetic contributors. While incurable, management strategies like medication, cognitive therapy, and lifestyle changes offer hope for symptom relief. Understanding these factors equips us to better support those affected and highlights the importance of ongoing research into prevention and treatment.

Chapter 7: Example of a mental health disorder: Stress and Anxiety

In this chapter, we discuss stress and anxiety, which are very common mental disorders that have a negative effect on one's mental health.

7.1 What is stress and anxiety

Stress is the subjective state of sensing potentially adverse changes in the environment that will lead to a response that enables the animal to adapt to the changing environment.

Anxiety is among the most frequent disorders in young people and most anxiety disorders originate in childhood.

The DSM-5 criteria for generalized anxiety disorder includes the following:

- restlessless
- fatigue
- difficulty in concentrating
- irritability
- muscle tension
- sleep disturbance associated with anxiety or worry, that the person finds difficult to control.

Anxiety occurs in a variety of forms including panic disorders and phobias, with young people being especially prone to social anxiety. Anxiety in childhood is associated with later risks of depression, substance abuse and suicidal behaviour.

7.2 Process of stress

Stress is a process with the following steps:

- The adverse changes in the environment are perceived by the brain regions, leading to release of stress mediator molecules to deal with the changes.
- This triggers the stress responses in the person, including physiological, cognitive and behavioral responses, that enable the person to adapt to the stressful changes in the environment.

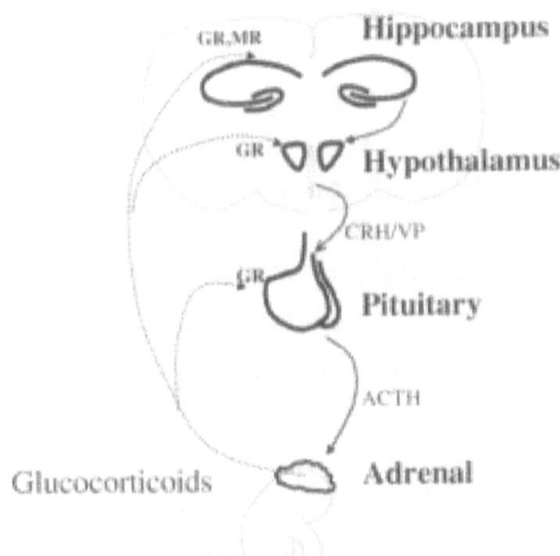

Figure: The hypothalamic-pituitary-adrenal (HPA) axis, that is activated by stress. Macedonian Academy of Sciences and Arts, CC BY-SA 4.0 <https://creativecommons.org/licenses/by-sa/4.0>, via Wikimedia Commons

7.3 Biology of stress

Stress is associated with activation of the HPA axis (hypothalamic–pituitary–adrenal axis) of the brain and spinal cord.

This involves the activation of the region of the brain called hypothalamus, which then activates the pituitary glands and then affects the adrenal cortex activating the adrenal glands.

The adrenal gland releases the hormone cortisol in the blood. This causes changes in the sympathetic nervous system, which governs the fight or flight response, causing changes such as pupil dilation, conversion of glycogen to glucose, secretion of adrenaline and noradrenaline, reduces the bladder constriction and digestive system, increases heart rate etc. It also causes changes in the immune system, cardiovascular system affecting blood pressure, and related changes, in such a way that one is better equipped to deal with the stressor.

This normal adaptive response is termed as allostasis.

Repeated, prolonged or chronic stress can reduce the effectiveness of the normal allostatic response of the body It can weaken our immune system, cause health conditions such as diabetes and significantly weaken our standard of life, this is called allostatic load.

Cortisol is the stress hormone, which is secreted by the HPA axis, stimulated by the prefrontal cortex and limbic system. Increased cortisol in the body results in increased blood pressure and heart rate, diverts resources away from inflammatory areas, weakening the immune system, and improves the memory and thinking. In the short term this is beneficial but in the long-term, chronic stress can cause a toxic build up.

7.4 Mindfulness for stress reduction

Mindfulness refers to purposefully paying attention to whatever arises in our awareness in the present moment, without reacting and non-judgmentally (Kabat-Zinn, 2015). Elements of mindfulness such as non-judgmentally observing thoughts, sensations and emotions in the present moment have benefits for mental health. Mindfulness has successfully been used to treat a number of mental health issues including anxiety among adolescents and others (Hofmann et al., 2010).

Mindfulness involves exercises such as sitting in a meditation posture and paying attention to the breath as it comes in and goes out through the nostrils.

In mindfulness practice, one pays gentle and sustained focused attention on the breath. If the mind wanders, such as a thought occurs or an itch or pain sensation occurs, one notices the sensation, and gently returns to noting the breath.

The mechanism of mindfulness is as follows: it is training to note our body sensations as they occur and thus increase our awareness of the stress response. It also trains us to accept our thoughts and feelings as they occur, without judging them as desirable or not.

Mindfulness can be practiced in both structured as well as unstructured forms. A common structured and well-studied form of mindfulness is an 8-week Structured program, called Mindfulness based Stress Reduction (MBSR). It was invented by Jon Kabat Zinn.

Mindfulness helps to enhance the immune system and other mechanisms.

Biological markers of stress include the cortisol levels in saliva and blood, blood pressure, heart rate variability, cytokine levels, and so on. These biological markers have been measured in various studies and confirmed to be improved by practicing mindfulness meditation.

7.5 Conclusion

In this chapter, we have discussed stress and anxiety as mental disorders, understood some of the biopsychosocial factors and explored mindfulness as a technique to control chronic stress.

In the next few chapters, we will go through some stress control techniques in more detail, since stress is very common, well-studied and directly impacts our well-being.

Chapter 8: Impact of diet and exercise on mental health

In this chapter, we discuss ways in which the food we eat our physical activity impacts our mental health.

8.1 Gut brain axis

The gut brain axis states that the brain and the gut (our digestive system including the stomach) are connected, and one affects the other. This connection is via the body's immune system and other systems such as nerve pathways and endocrine system.

A good state of the gut can, therefore, result in better mental health and lack of mental diseases and disorders. On the other hand, imbalances in our gut bacteria, caused due to factors such as diet and also environment, genetics and other factors, can lead to depression or anxiety. Therefore, we need to make sure that our diet is well balanced and diverse, and follows good diet guidelines.

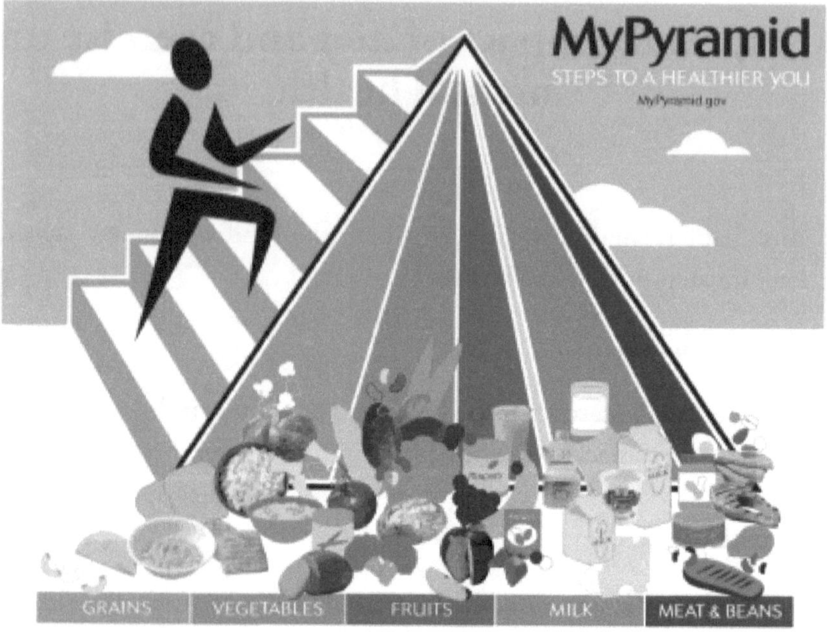

Figure: The USDA's food pyramid, suggesting the breakdown of a healthy diet, MyPyramid. By United States Department of Agriculture - http://www.mypyramid.gov, Public Domain, https://commons.wikimedia.org/w/index.php?curid=12811268

8.2 World Health Organization guidelines on diet

Among the world health organization (WHO) recommendations for a healthy diet are the following:

(from https://www.who.int/health-topics/healthy-diet)

- Have a varied diet, largely plant based, and balance your energy intake with expenditure of calories.
- Obtaining the largest amount of energy from carbohydrates, mainly through legumes, lentils, beans and wholegrain cereals.
- Reducing total fats to less than 30% of total energy intake,

shifting fat intake away from saturated and trans fat to unsaturated fats.

- Reducing free sugars to less than 10% of total energy intake, including reducing sugary drinks.
- Limiting sodium intake to less than 2 gms per day (which is 5 grams or one tablespoon of salt).
- Consuming at least 400 grams of vegetables and fruit per day in adults.

Following these good and healthy diet practices, such as increasing the variety and amount of plant based foods such as fresh fruit and veggies and decreasing processed foods and meat as well as salt and sugar intake, can result in a healthy diet and consequently a better mental health for us.

8.3 Moderate physical activity

WHO also recommends moderate physical activity and exercise every day, which can also improve one's mental well-being. This can include walking, jogging, cycling, dancing, yoga or other exercise, swimming or some sport involving physical activity.

8.4 Conclusion

In this chapter, we have briefly discussed the importance of good diet and physical activity towards cultivating good mental health.

Chapter 9: Techniques for Dealing with Stress

In this chapter, we discuss the ways in which this stress can affect us and ways in which we can deal with it in the short term.

9.1 The Stress Cycle

The definition of stress as per the World Health Organization is as follows: *"Stress is the reaction people may have when presented with demands and pressures that are not matched to their knowledge and abilities and which challenge their ability to cope."*

Stress normally works in a cycle. The cycle works as follows:

- We may get stressed because of a variety of factors
- Because of stress, we can manifest different kinds of reactions. We may turn to overeating or alcohol to deal with the stress. Stress may lead to bodily symptoms such as increased heart rate, short breaths, high blood pressure, diabetes, indigestion and so on. We can become more prone to negative emotions such as anger. Our behavior may become moody and unpredictable and fluctuating. Our ability to function socially might become worse and we may become withdrawn from our friends and relatives. We may indulge in negative self-talk such as thinking that we are worthless or failures. We may become less able to concentrate and more prone to get distracted.
- All these could lead to worse effects such as heart diseases, mental illnesses, affect our memory and sleep, cause premature aging and so on.
- This could lead to lesser enjoyment and productivity in life,

leading to even greater stress.

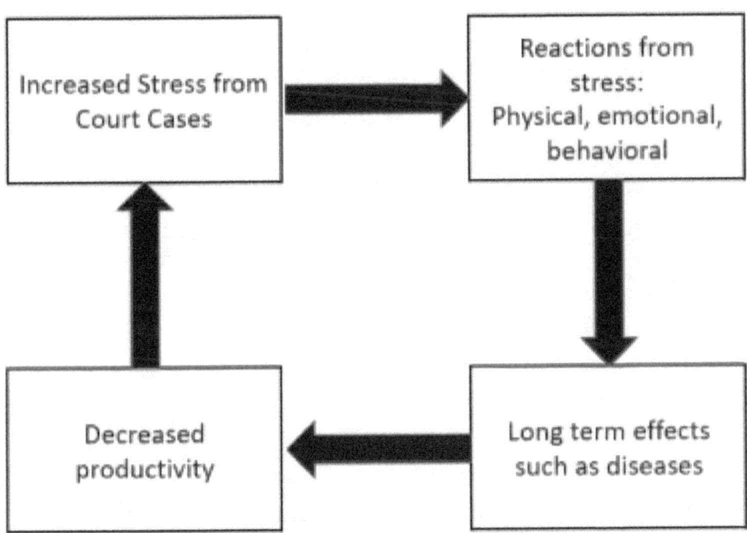

Figure: Illustration of the stress cycle

This stress cycle goes on and on, increasing our stress and further decreasing our ability to deal with our everyday tasks.

9.2 Systematic ways to tackle stress

In order to tackle stress and break the stress cycle, we can follow a few simple steps, which are as follows:

- We should aim to have regular meals and good sleep.
- We should aim to keep active including a regular exercise schedule. For example, we can do a few simple yoga exercises, such as a few cycles of "surya namaskara" yoga exercise.
- We should cultivate some hobbies to keep our brain active.
- We should make it a point to keep meeting our close friends and well-wishers.
- We should try not to indulge in negative thoughts such as

obsessing about the case and hypothetical situations or blaming others for our problems. We should also not try to control everything.

- We should try and balance our time, keeping adequate me-time for ourselves as well as allocate enough time for our family.

By following all the above steps, we would be able to improve our mental health and be stronger and better able to deal with stressful situations.

9.3 Simple techniques to combat stress

We can check ourselves from time to time if we are having the symptoms of stress such as short breaths, shallow breaths, slumped posture and so on.

If we detect that our breath and posture are showing signs of stress, we can follow a few simple techniques to come out of stress in the short term, which are discussed in the following subsections.

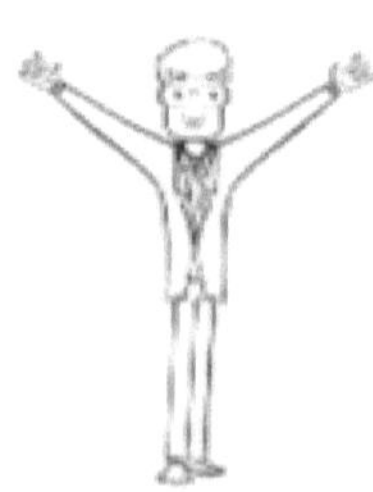
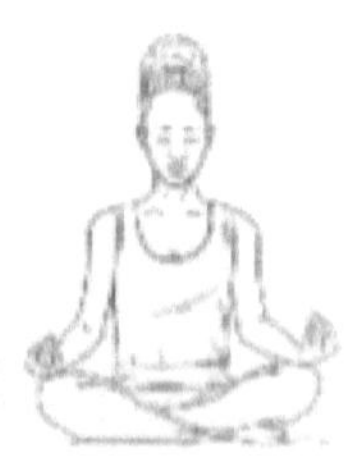

Figure: Steps for combating stress

9.3.1 Longer and slower breaths

When we are stressed, our breathing becomes very shallow and short and fast. Therefore, one technique to control stress can be to consciously make our breath longer and deeper, make sure our breath is slower and reaches all the way till the stomach. This technique has the immediate effect of lowering our stress level. Same goes for the posture and body language: having an upright posture and a positive body language can also play a role in lowering our stress levels.

9.3.2 Mindfulness meditation

Another technique for lowering stress can be to follow mindfulness meditation for a few minutes daily. This involves sitting with our back straight, closing our eyes, mindfully observing the various sensations of our body slowly from head to toe, and counting each breath.

We can count the breaths by silently counting from 1 to 10 with each inbreath, and again restarting at 1 after the cycle of 10 breaths is completed.

9.3.3 Smiling more

One way to beat stress can be simply to smile more. The act of smiling tricks our brain into believing we are happy and relaxed, and the body also exhibits the symptoms of relaxation rather than stress.

9.3.4 Reframing and keeping a positive attitude

Another way to combat stress is to keep a positive attitude. This can be done in the following ways:

- Every morning we can bring to mind all the things we are grateful for, all the people who have helped us and are helping us in our life.
- We can make positive affirmations such as *"may myself and others be happy and well"*, and *"may all the people around us also*

be happy and well".

- We can try to mentally forgive people we perceive have harmed us, as well as any others we may be having grudges against.
- We can encourage ourselves with positive self-talk encouraging ourselves, as opposed to negative self-talk.
- We can think of the adversity almost as a test of our patience and a training for us to become mentally stronger.
- We can use this opportunity to think of other people who are caught in similar adverse situations as us, empathize with them and wish them well.
- We can take the opportunity to help people around us in ways big and small, which has the side effect of improving our own mental health and relieving our own stress.

By following the above steps regularly and sustained over a period of time, we might be able to combat stress effectively and start a "wellness cycle" that can fight the stress cycle.

9.4 Cultivating a carefree attitude in life

One way to reduce our stress and more generally is to cultivate a carefree attitude to whatever happens in our life. We should not always try to control everything or expect things to go well. The whole of our life is a learning process, and we should be aware of this.

In order to cultivate this attitude, we should not be unduly concerned with what is happening or what others may be thinking of us. We should make it a habit to take some time off for ourselves, take regular breaks from work and commitments, and take regular walks and retreats in the midst of nature.

We should also endeavor to cultivate a child-like inquisitive mind no matter what our age, since it helps our brain to continue making new connections, become more efficient and think of different out of the box and creative ways to deal with our problems.

9.5 Conclusion

In this chapter, we have looked at some practical ways and means to get relief from stress, at least in the short term.

Chapter 10: Using the Cognitive Model and CBT to Control Negative Thoughts

In the earlier chapters we have suggested a few mechanisms to reduce stress and related symptoms.

In this chapter we look at the cognitive model of psychotherapy and explore how it can be used to better handle adverse and stressful situations by controlling the negative thoughts that may arise.

10.1 The cognitive model

A famous American psychologist named Aaron Beck introduced the cognitive model of psychology in 1960s. As per this model, our thoughts affect our behavior and feelings. Hence, to deal with stress, one key aspect is to examine our thoughts and beliefs and assumptions and understand how they are affecting our feelings and behavior.

Beck's cognitive model (Beck, 1967) comprises a triad of automatic negative thoughts or schemas by the subject, that includes dysfunctional thoughts about themselves, the world and the future. These schemas are often formed by earlier experiences in one's life, may be latent but get activated by adverse events in one's environment.

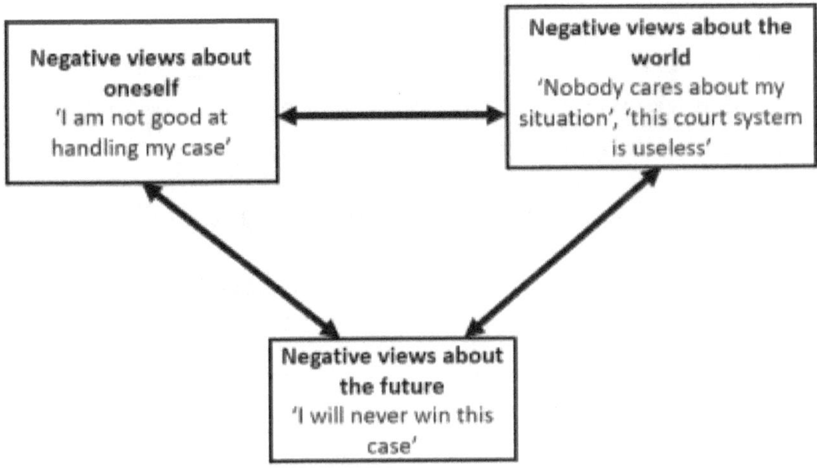

Figure: Illustration about the cognitive triad, how negative thoughts about oneself, the world and future feed into each other

One of the ways this works is via the cognitive triad as shown in the figure above. This comprises the following:

- We have negative thoughts about ourselves
- We have negative thoughts about the world
- We have negative thoughts about the future

These negative views and thoughts feed into each other and create a spiral of ever more negative thinking. This can adversely affect our health and well-being.

For example, a subject may have failed or performed badly in an academic test, leading to negative thoughts such as:

'I do not deserve to pass this course' (negative thought about themselves)

'this course is too complicated to understand' (negative thought about the world)

'I shall never be able to pass this course' (negative thought about the future).

The subjects may also have cognitive distortions or biases in their thinking that lead them to pay selective attention to the negative aspects of situations, while ignoring any positive aspects.

Some examples of such cognitive distortions include the following:

- overgeneralization (making a generalized conclusion or inference based on only a few events)
- selective abstraction (drawing conclusions about the situation on the basis of just a tiny bit of evidence)
- magnification (focusing on the negative aspects of the situation)
- minimization (downplaying the positive aspects of the situation)
- personalization (blaming oneself for causing the situation, to the exclusion of other factors).

These biases result in a pessimistic explanatory style, through which the depressed persons view and explain everything through a pessimistic lens. All of these factors together maintain the cycle of negative thoughts that may cause the subject to remain in a state of depression or drive episodes of depression.

The way out is to understand how this negative cycle of thoughts really works, and then try to combat the same using positive thoughts and questioning our negative assumptions that may not be grounded in reality.

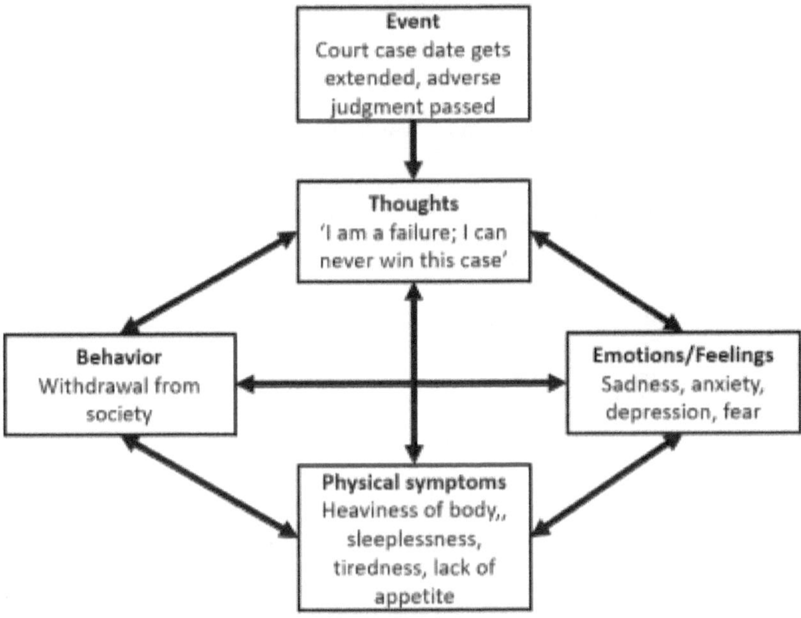

Figure: Illustration about how negative events can affect our feelings, thoughts, physical symptoms and behavior, as per the cognitive model in psychology

10.2 Understanding the link between behavior, thinking and emotions

As per the cognitive model in psychology, there is a link between our thinking, emotions, physical sensations and behavior and these feed upon each other.

For example, the following is an example:

External event: An external event can be an adverse incident that happened that day.

This external event can produce the following:

- **Negative thoughts**: Thoughts such as "I will never win this case", "This case is going on so long without any result", "I am worthless"
- **Feelings and emotions**: These include sadness, fear, anxiety, depression.
- **Physical sensations**: These include heaviness in the body, lack of sleep, lack of appetite.

This in turn can lead to the following:

Behaviors: Resulting behaviors can include reduced contact with others, feeling withdrawn, sitting in one place, lying in bed till late in the day and so on.

If this continues for a period of time, mental health conditions such as depression and anxiety, and health issues such as diabetes can result.

This is the way in which negative thoughts can lead to negative feelings and conditions like depression. We should understand the way in which these factors are interlinked. Understanding this will help us to form a strategy to break the cycle.

10.3 Using CBT (Cognitive Behavior Therapy) and challenging negative thoughts

Cognitive Behavior Therapy (CBT) was developed by Aaron Beck in 1960s and 1970s and provides a structured framework and therapy to break the cycle of negative thoughts. It has been successfully used all over the world in cases of depression, anxiety and other conditions. It follows methods to break the cycle of negative thoughts and cultivate more realistic appraisals of unfavorable situations.

To use CBT, one can either see a counsellor who is qualified in CBT or consults books and videos on its methods.

Once we understand the cognitive model as to how negative thoughts cause negative feelings and lead to unhelpful behaviors, we can take actions to challenge our negative thoughts and gradually replace them with positive thoughts. The challenge is to break the negative cycle and link, and for this the method is to question our hidden core beliefs behind our negative thoughts (such as 'I am worthless') using logic and evidence from our past experiences.

For this, we should carefully note our momentary thoughts when we have negative emotions. We can then analyze the thoughts in order to understand the root of those thoughts. Once we have written them down, we should examine how or why such thoughts are coming and challenge ourselves with the opposite evidence.

An example of this can be as follows: If we have an unfavorable event, we may think that it is our fault and that we are worthless. In actuality, the unfavorable event could be due to reasons beyond our control. In such a case, we should challenge our negative thoughts instead of ruminating on them. We should bring to mind the times when we had successfully handled similar and more challenging situations in life. Therefore, it is incorrect to think that we cannot handle such situations or that we are a failure simply because we were unlucky to get one unfavorable event.

10.4 Cultivating positive thoughts and activities

Since we are often prone to focusing unduly on the negative thoughts, one remedy can be to instead focus on our positive thoughts and experiences deliberately.

We can recall our achievements in life, thinking of instances where we have been successfully handling our job and family in the past.

By repeatedly recalling and training our mind to focus on the positive aspects and using this to challenge our recurring negative thoughts, we can break the cycle of negativity and gain freedom from stress, anxiety and depression.

We can also schedule some physical activities during the day to break out from the mold of brooding about the case. We can try things like walking, exercise, gym, and standing during work or moving frequently rather than sitting on a chair for long periods.

10.5 Using Mindfulness along with CBT and positive thoughts

Mindfulness is a way of bringing our notice to the immediate thoughts and feelings at each moment, with a feeling of acceptance to whatever is going on and without being judgmental. The most common way to practice mindfulness is to close our eyes and calmly turn our attention to the thoughts, feelings and sensations in the mind and all parts of the body.

One can practice mindfulness in one of these two ways:

- Do a body scan, going systematically from top of the head till the feet, and pay attention to the sensations and feelings from each part systematically.
- Just let the mind free, do not dwell on the thoughts. Bring attention to whichever sensations or feelings are the strongest at that moment.

Mindfulness practice involves cultivating a feeling of acceptance to whatever is happening without thinking too much about it. Using mindfulness with each sensation or thought or feeling, we remain in the present moment without judgment, just mindfully acknowledge the thought and let it go. Adding mindfulness to CBT means using the CBT methods and cultivating an added feeling of acceptance to the thoughts as they come and go without getting too involved in them and getting caught up in a spiral of the negative thoughts.

Even when we are suffering from health or financial issues, we can mindfully notice each negative thought as it comes, acknowledge it without dwelling on it and just let it go and return to mindfulness of the body and other sensations.

This practice can be done on a regular basis for a few minutes every day. Once we have gained familiarity with this practice, it can help us to better deal with the negative cycle of thoughts and feelings as we discussed earlier.

10.6 Conclusion

In this chapter we have learnt about the cognitive model that explains how our thoughts are linked to feelings and behaviors. We have also discussed the ways by which we can combine the benefits of mindfulness with the CBT techniques of understanding the relation between thoughts and feelings, questioning our negative thoughts and focusing on positive thoughts and experiences.

By applying all these techniques to our negative feelings and thoughts, we can effectively manage stress, anxiety and depression that arise from such difficult situations.

Chapter 11: Some CBT based apps for mental health

In this chapter, we discuss a few good apps using Cognitive Behavioral Therapy (CBT) and related therapies, that are useful for promotion of mental health.

11.1 List of well-being apps based on CBT

A few good CBT apps for well-being, are as follows:

- Wysa
- Calm harm
- Move mood
- SAM
- What's up
- Mindshift

In the sections below, we go through each of these apps in more detail.

11.2 Wysa

Wysa is a chatbot based on CBT. It is almost like a virtual therapist. It is approved by the NHS (National Health Service) as part of mental health treatments in UK.

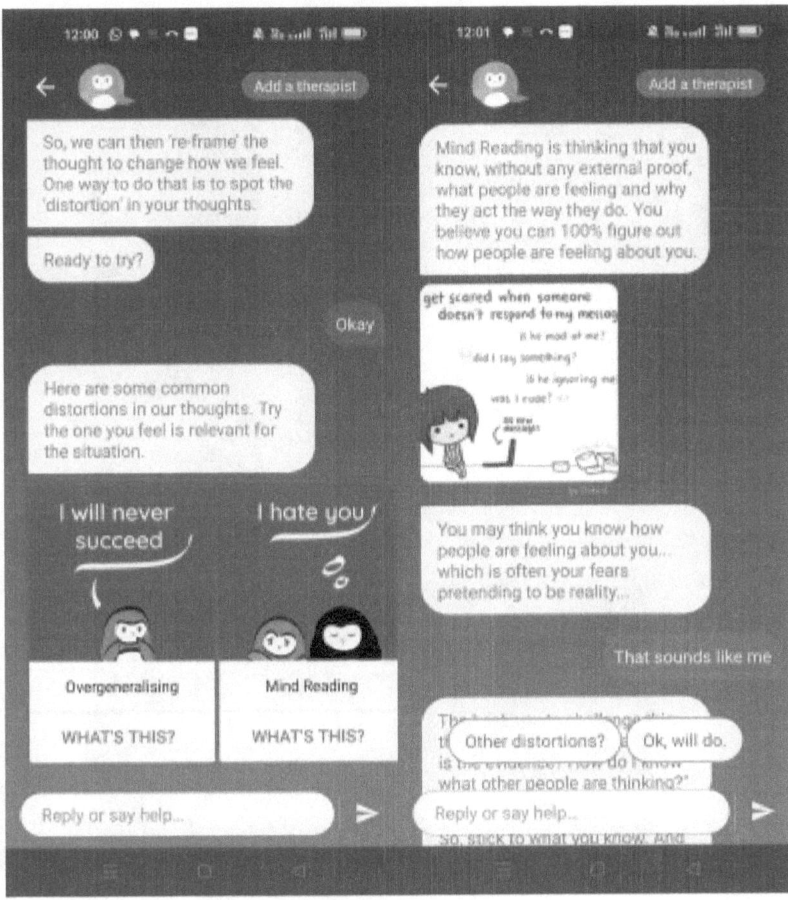

Figure: Screenshots of Wysa chatbot app

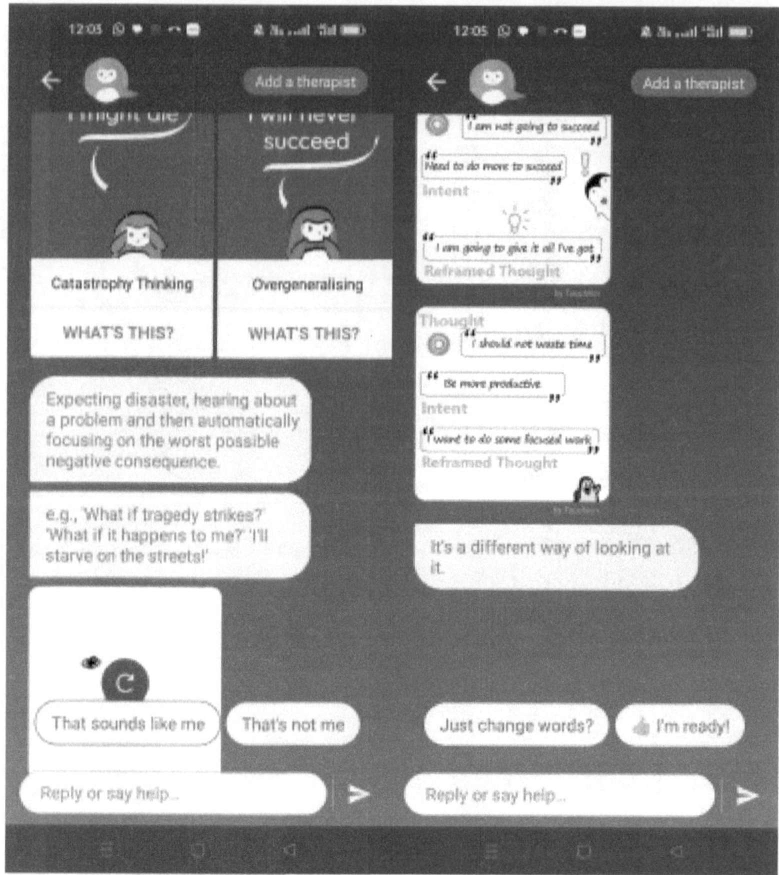

Figure: Screenshots of Wysa chatbot app

Its website is: https://www.wysa.com/nhs

Wysa functions as a friendly and confidential chatbot with whom we can have a conversation, let them know what is worrying us. The chatbot suggests solutions in a calm and empathetic way. It also links to guided meditations for anxiety and other problems. The guided meditations etc are started on the user's mobile as part of the chatbot app.

11.3 Calm harm

Calm harm is an app to resist self-harm and unhelpful thoughts. It is based on principles of DBT or dialectical behavior therapy. The idea is that thoughts of self-harm do not arise suddenly, they are part of a chain of thoughts and strong emotions, a bit like riding a wave of emotions. If the user is aware of such thoughts and emotions when they arise, this chain can be broken.

It has several features such as an activity log, recording how we are feeling or what activities we are doing any time of the day. It also suggests many kinds of activities one can do if we are feeling negative thoughts or feel the urge to self-harm.

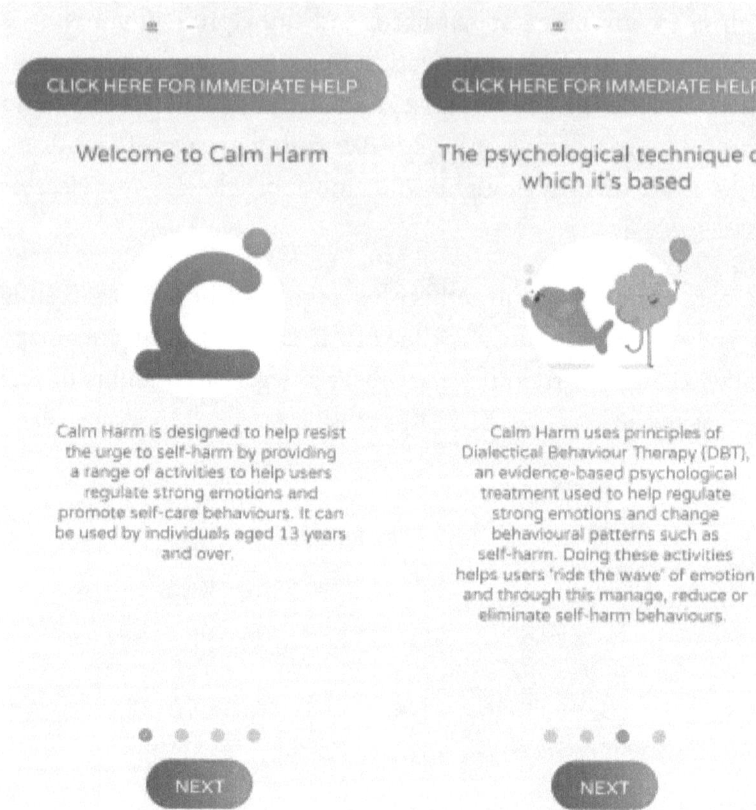

Figure: Screenshots of Calm Harm app

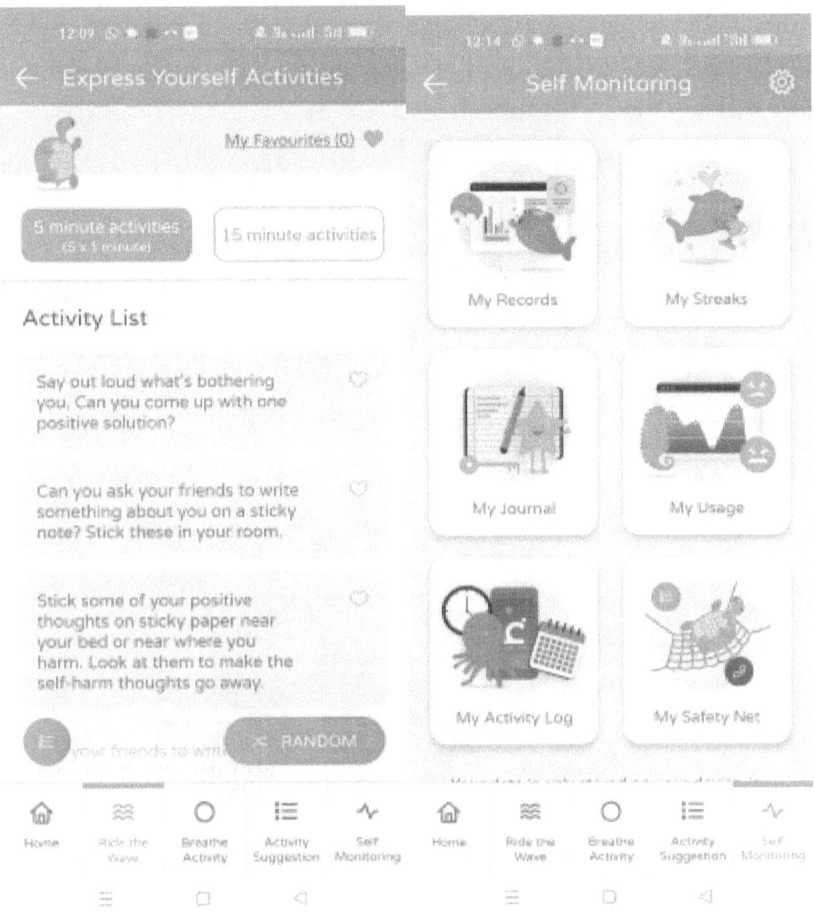

Figure: Screenshots of Calm Harm app

11.4 Move mood

Move Mood is an app to manage low moods and depression. It is based on Behavioral Activation Therapy, setting daily tasks to come out of low moods.

The idea is that when one is feeling depressed or in a low mood, doing small tasks that are fun or meaningful can enable the user to come out of such moods, or "move" the mood.

The website of the app is https://movemood.stem4.org.uk/

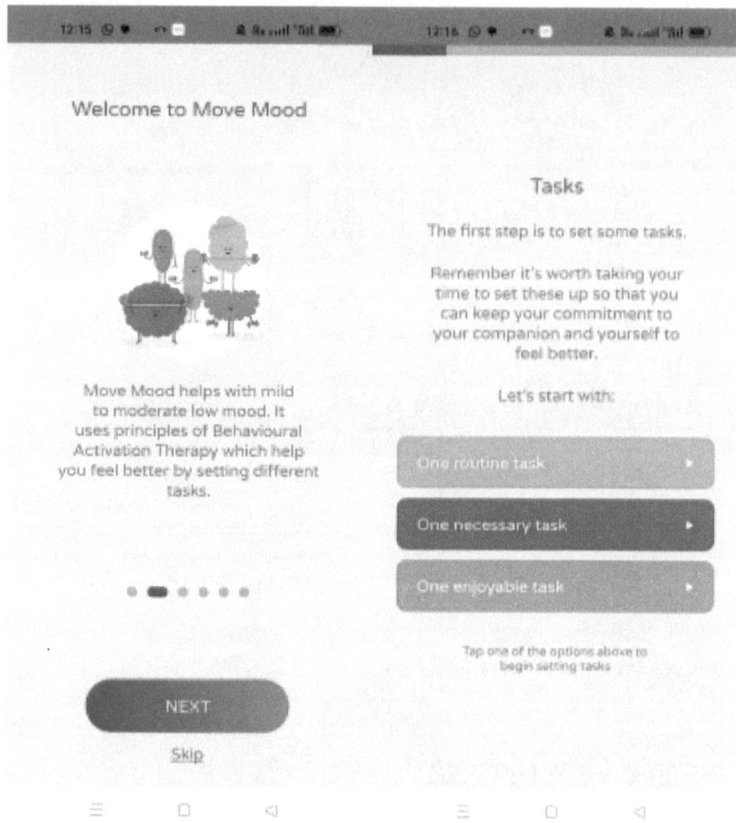

Figure: Screenshots of Move Mood app

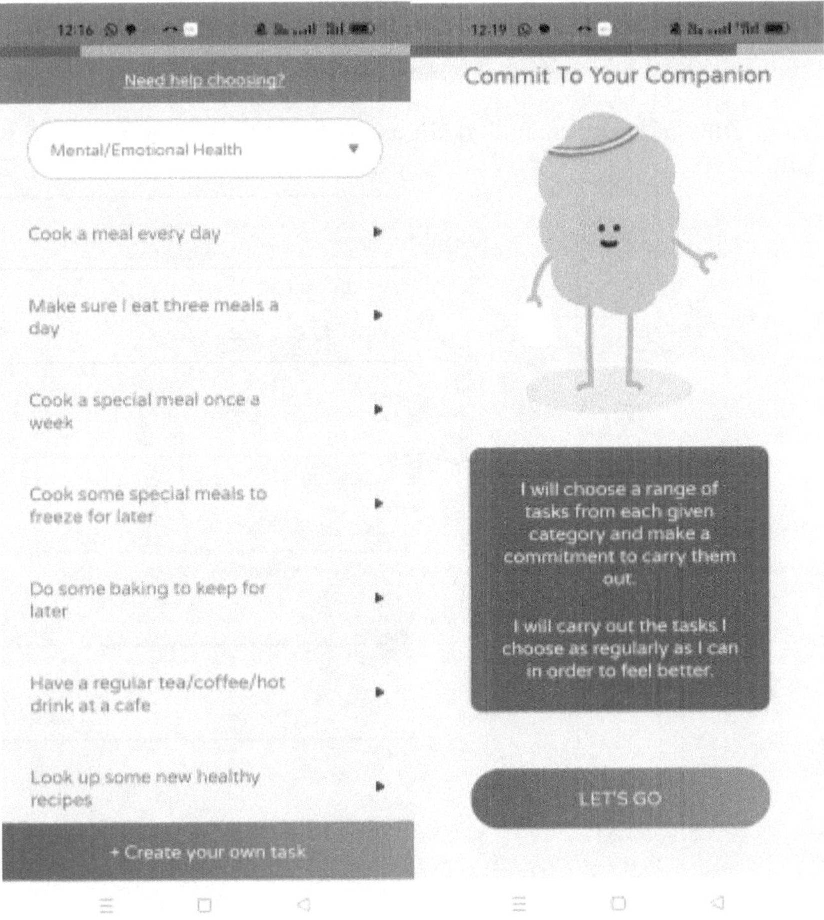

Figure: Screenshots of Move Mood app

This link gives more information on how behavioral activation can help: https://www.webmd.com/mental-health/behavioral-activation-how-to-use-it

11.5 SAM app

SAM is a self-help app for the mind. It is an app to manage anxiety, depression and loneliness. The user can themselves use it, with or without the help of a supporting therapist, to manage their own mental health issues. It is backed by academic research as well.

It has a series of features and meditations for different issues such as anxiety.

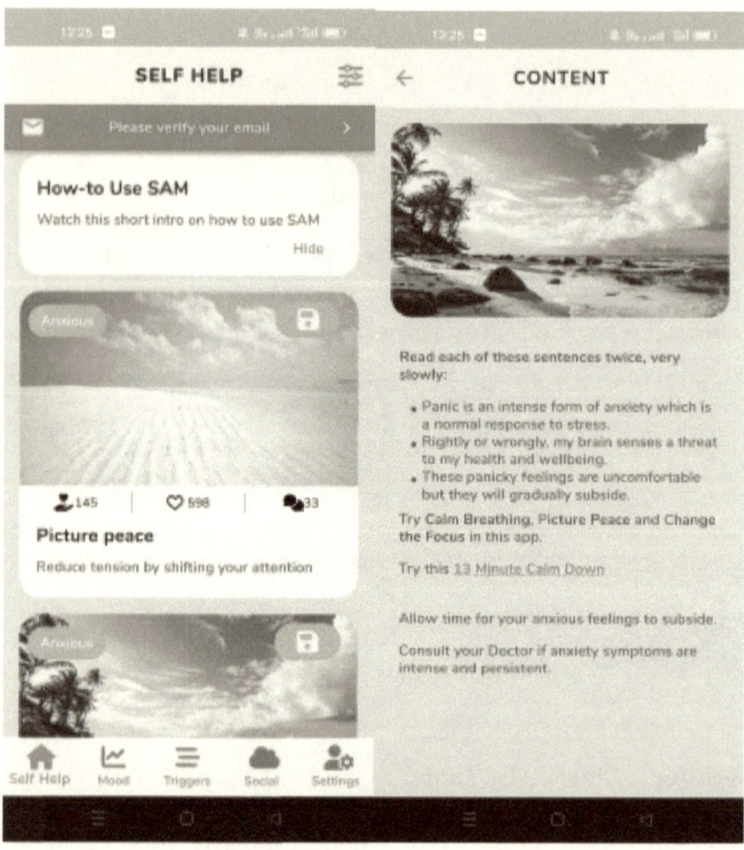

Figure: Screenshots of SAM app

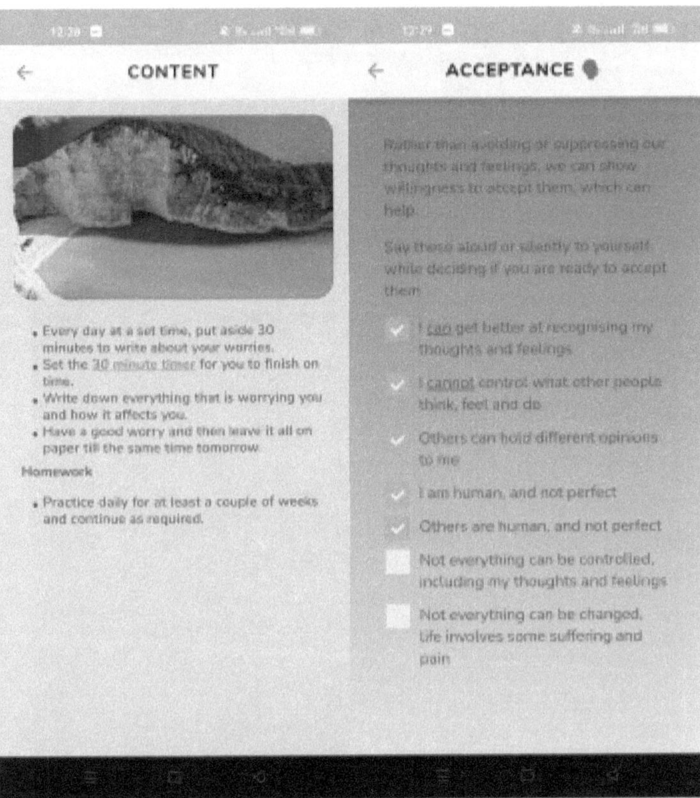

Figure: Screenshots of SAM app

The website of the SAM app is as follows: mindgarden-tech.co.uk

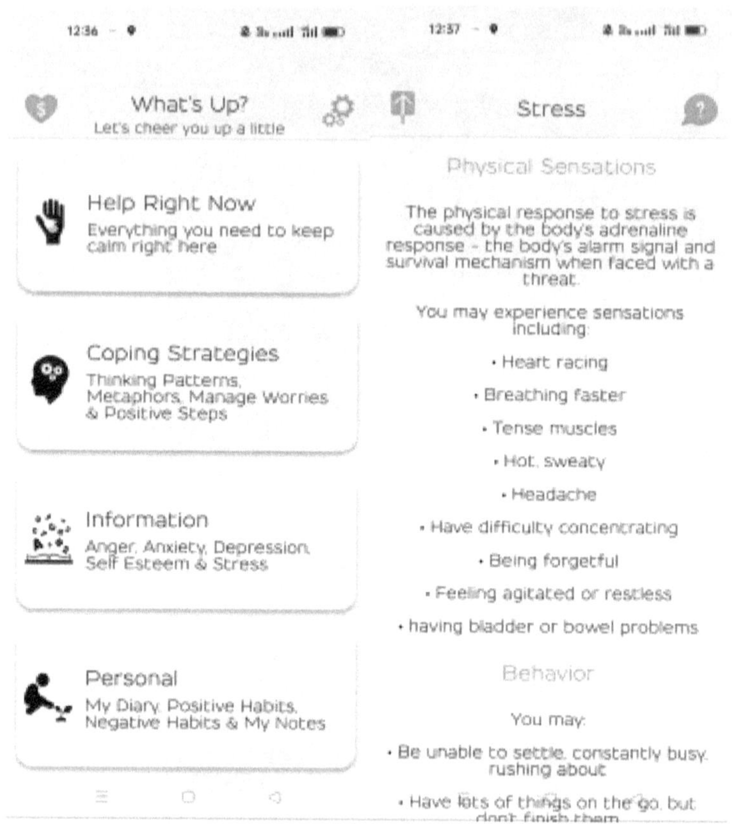

Figure: Screenshots of What's Up app

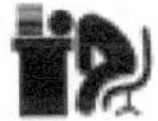

Figure: Screenshots of What's Up app

11.6 What's up

What's up is an app to promote one's own mental health. It has features like rating one's own mood at different times of the day, a directory of wellbeing contacts, and steps for wellbeing.

The website of What's up app is as follows: www.thewhatsupapp.co.uk[1]

---

1. http://www.thewhatsupapp.co.uk/

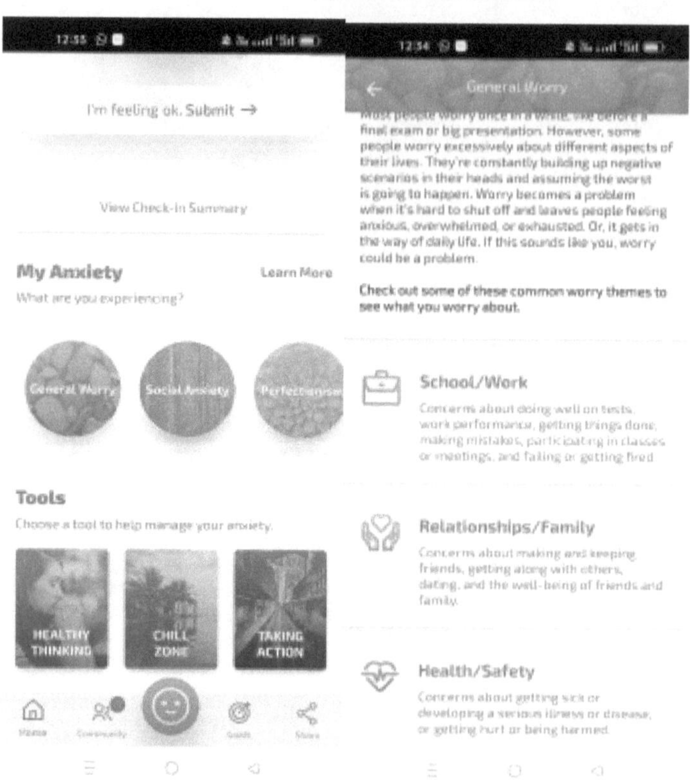

Figure: Screenshots of Mindshift app

11.7 Mindshift

Mindshift is an app to manage anxiety, based on CBT. It has a lot of information on how negative thinking patterns cause anxiety and other conditions, and what an user can do to come out of unhelpful thought patterns. It also has a section on different types of coping strategies.

The website of the Mindshift app is https://www.anxietycanada.com/resources/mindshift-cbt/

11.8 Conclusion

In this article, we have briefly discussed some of the free and useful well-being apps related to CBT. Each of these apps have their own specialties, based on different aspects of CBT and its variants, and are useful for different types of mental health issues in different users. The user can install these on their own mobile devices. They function as a source of additional support for one's well-being.

Chapter 12: Courses and apps related to mindfulness and well-being

In this chapter, we discuss a few good courses, books and apps based on mindfulness and other techniques, that can help with our mental health and well-being.

12.1 Mental health and well-being related courses

A good free online course on happiness and well-being is the "Science of Well-Being" at Coursera. It is one of the most popular courses at Coursera and has been taken by thousands of students.

The course is led by Laurie Santos at Yale. It has some basic theory of well-being, as well as practical strategies, based on scientific evidence, to enhance one's well-being and happiness. It goes through some misconceptions and biases we have about well-being, and discusses strategies to enhance it.

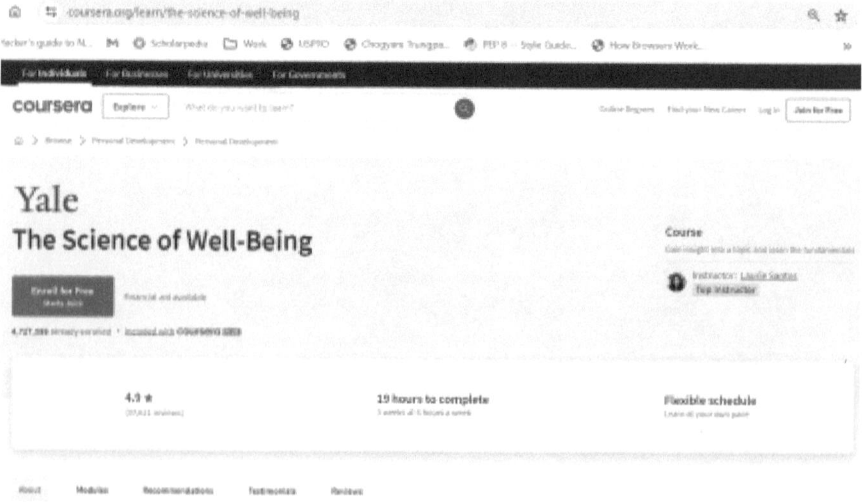

Figure: Screenshot of the Science of Well being app on Coursera

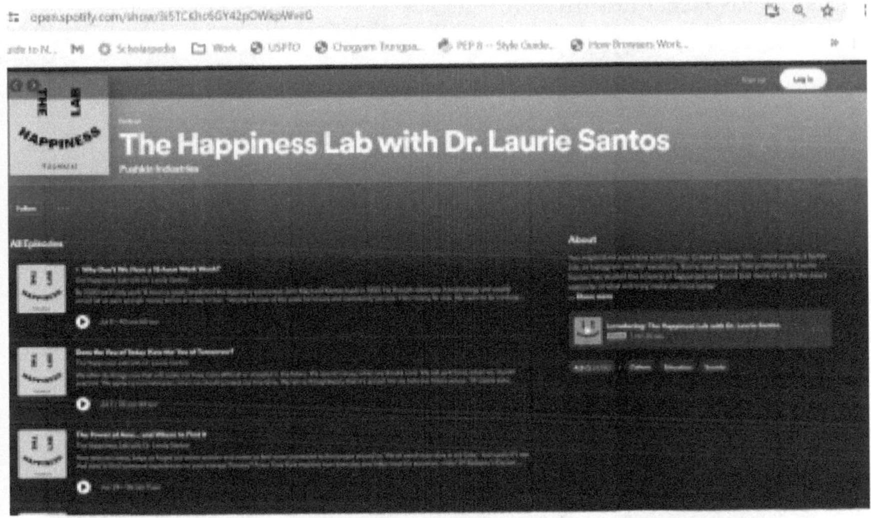

Figure: Screenshot of the Happiness Lab podcast on Spotify

Link to the Science of Well Being course on Coursera: https://www.coursera.org/learn/the-science-of-well-being

A related podcast on wellbeing is called the Happiness Lab with Laurie Santos, available on amazon audible and spotify. The link is https://open.spotify.com/show/3i5TCKhc6GY42pOWkpWveG

12.2 Mindfulness and other apps on mental health and well-being

Well-being enhancing apps include mindfulness apps, creativity apps, gratitude journal apps and CBT apps.

Mindfulness apps

There are a number of good mindfulness and meditation apps on the google play store or app store that can help us to do mindfulness meditation and enhance our feeling of well-being.

Examples are calm, insight timer, the mindfulness app, stop breathe and think, headspace, buddhify etc.

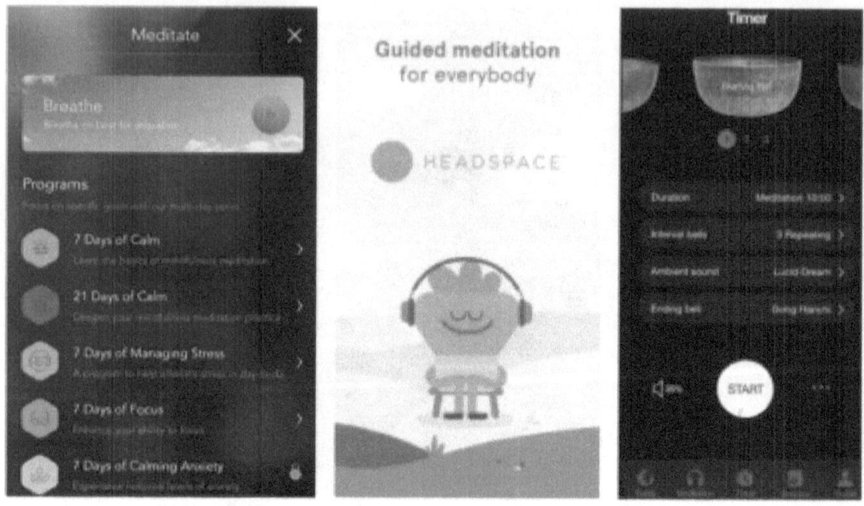

Figure: Some popular mindfulness meditation apps: Calm, Headspace, Insight Timer

The plum village website (https://plumvillage.org/mindfulness-practice/mindful-apps/) has a good number of useful links to mindful apps and related software.

However, it can become a problem if we install too many mindfulness apps! So it is better to try them out, choose a few (maximum 4 or 5) that we like best, then uninstall the other apps.

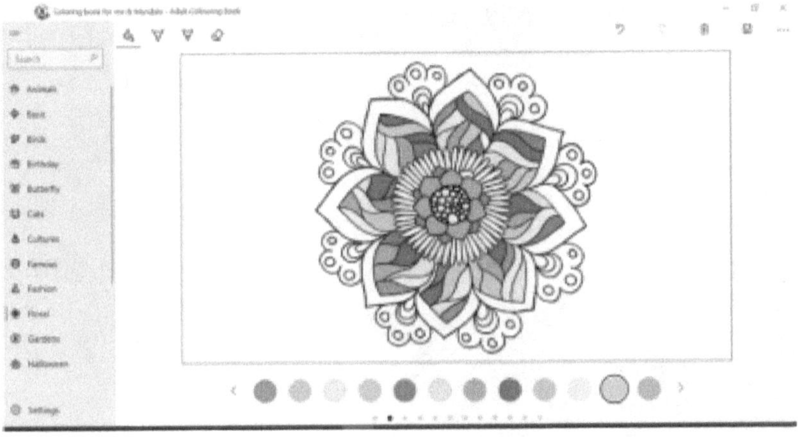

Figure: Screenshot of a mandala colouring app, downloaded from the Windows store

Using creativity enhancing apps

Examples of creativity enhancing apps include mindfulness coloring apps. While using coloring apps, our mindfulness can be cultivated since we are focused on coloring and not distracted by thoughts.

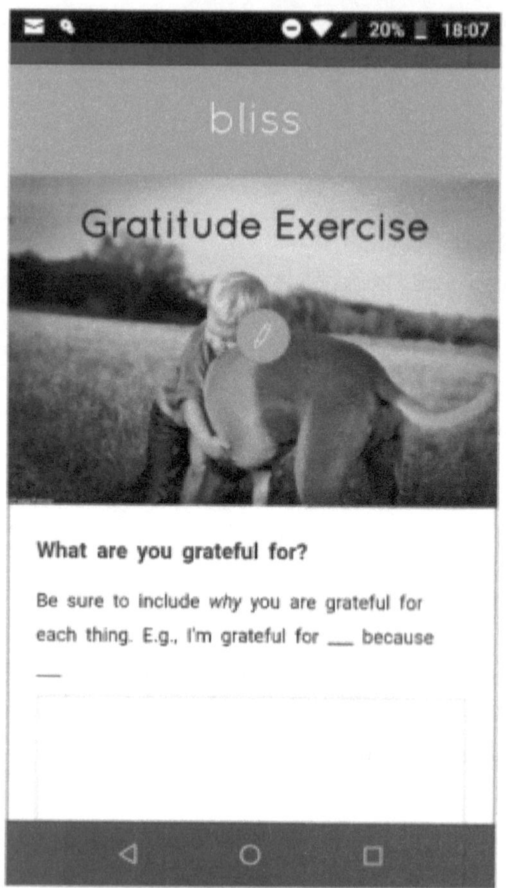

Figure: Screenshot of a gratitude exercise on Bliss, a happiness journal app

Using gratitude journal apps

Research has shown that expressing gratitude and remembering what we are thankful for can go a long way towards enhancing our sense of well-being. Many apps are available that help one to keep a daily gratitude journal or use other positive psychology tools to enhance happiness. Some of these apps are Reimagining the examen, track your happiness, Bliss, and gratitude journal. These apps are a great complement to any other meditation apps you may have, to fill in during the day or before going to bed. Daily reminding ourselves what we are grateful for and going through how the day went and positive experiences we had throughout the day can trick the brain into feeling happier.

Using happiness related apps

A good happiness enhancing app is Happify.

Another good happiness app is called the Happiness Project.

Both of these can be downloaded from the google play store or apple app store.

12.3 Conclusion

In this chapter, we have briefly discussed a few online courses and apps to enhance our happiness and well-being, including mindfulness apps, gratitude journals and happiness apps.

Chapter 13: Using Behavioral Therapy to Control Anxiety and Worry

In this chapter, we discuss some techniques from behavioral therapy to help with anxiety and worry while facing difficult, stressful or anxiety inducing situations.

13.1 Introduction to conditioning and behavioral therapy

Behavioral therapy aims to modify one's behavior using methods such as classical conditioning and operant conditioning to reinforce our desired behavior (not having stress) and decrease the negative or undesired behavior (such as feeling stressed or anxious).

Conditioning involves training a person to pair a desired **stimulus** with a desired **response** or **behavior**. The technique was first studied and developed by a Russian psychologist named Ivan Pavlov in the 19th century, who trained a dog to pair the sound of a bell and the dog's salivation expecting food when the bell was rung.

A common type of conditioning is called operant conditioning. It includes the skillful use of punishment and reinforcement as a way to increase or decrease certain behaviors to cultivate more desirable ones.

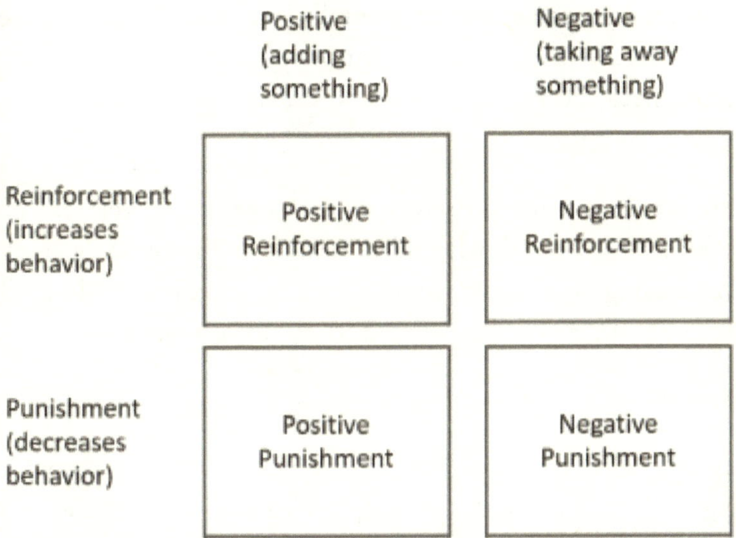

Figure: Illustration of operant conditioning

13.2 Application of conditioning to anxiety

Many times, we may feel scared, stressed or anxious, dreading what might happen when the stressful situation arises. This kind of stress reaction might be automatic, considering that we do not have control over the situation. This loss of control can make us feel uncomfortable.

One way to control such anxiety is to train ourselves to **pair** the stressful situation with something **pleasant**, such as a happy memory or music we like. This can be done by consciously recalling the happy memory or playing our favorite music each time, we have the feeling of being stressed or anxious. This would train our brain to associate the next date with something pleasant instead of unpleasant.

13.3 Training to acclimatize to the stressful situations using exposure

Another way is to gradually train ourselves to control our fear and stress in real life situations using gradual exposure. This can be done, for example, by recreating the situation mentally and visualizing how we can deal with it in a relaxed way. This can help us to become familiar with the atmosphere and to train not to be stressed by exposure to the non-threatening condition.

In addition, we can train ourselves to become more relaxed by consciously breathing more slowly and deeply, having a confident body language and smiling more when facing a stressful situation. Such small actions trick our brain into feeling of relaxed and lowers our stress.

13.4 Conclusion

In this chapter, we have discuss how to use behavioral therapy, with conditioning and reinforcement, to help us to deal with stress and stressful situations.

Chapter 14: Using Logotherapy to Find Higher Meaning in Stressful Situations

In this chapter, we consider logotherapy, a kind of therapy, as a means to finding higher meaning and purpose while facing stressful situations in life.

14.1 Introduction to logotherapy

The famous psychologist Viktor Frankl in his book "Man's Search for Meaning" proposed a way to deal with situations in life that cause suffering.

His theory was inspired by his own life experience and suffering of being imprisoned in the concentration camps by the Nazis during the holocaust in World War 2. He carefully observed how some inmates of the camps were able to survive the seemingly hopeless situation by thinking of it as only an intermediate step to achieving a higher goal or realizing a higher meaning in the future life. Those who could not visualize a higher meaning or future gave up and could not survive the experience of the concentration camps.

Frankl's insight was that as long as we can find some meaning or higher purpose in our suffering, it becomes easier for us to deal with it and bear the suffering.

This theory can be applied to dealing with all kinds of stressful situations.

14.2 Applying logotherapy to find higher meaning in stressful situations

We can use the principles of logotherapy to find higher meaning when facing adverse or stressful situations. As per logotherapy, meaning in life can be found in multiple ways, some of which are as follows:

- Self-awareness and self-discovery
- Finding meaning through work
- Finding meaning through hobbies
- Experiencing love: experiences with friends, family and people in social networks
- Developing a positive attitude
- Finding higher meaning in whatever work one is involved: the higher goal
- Cultivating resilience and fighting spirit when faced with adversity

Although the suffering might seem heavy when we are facing it, we should reflect on what can we learn from it and what is the deeper meaning of all this suffering for us. In this sense, it is like a tough teacher for us. But we do gain something from the experience.

We should reflect on how it can teach us to fight and be stronger no matter what life's difficulties are. Eventually one day, the situation will be over, and we can look forward to that day. We will then remember how we fought hard for what we believed in, despite all the suffering.

14.3 Conclusion

In this chapter we have considered how logotherapy can be used to find higher meaning and purpose in stressful situations. This can help us to cultivate a more positive attitude and combat negative thoughts.

Chapter 15: Forming a Support Group

In this chapter, we discuss another important way to deal with stress and improving our mental health, which is forming a support group of like-minded people who are dealing with similar situations and with whom we can share updates.

15.1 Benefits of forming a support group

There are many benefits of forming a self-help support group of like-minded people.

People in the group can get companionship and comradeship by helping each other. One can get strength from the fact that they are not alone and that there are others in similar situations. Negative emotions and stress can be reduced by the positive action of helping each other. One can also, depending on time, accompany each other and thus provide tangible encouragement and support.

15.2 How to form a support group

The first step in forming a support group is to find other people who are fighting similar situations. One can talk to other people, or from common friends find out about other people in the similar situations.

The next step is to organize a regular get-together or at least a common communication medium such as a WhatsApp chat group for mutual support.

The process of forming a group can be slower and a bit difficult initially, but as the number of people increase, it can get easier to run the group and make it self-sustaining. Therefore, it is worth putting the extra effort to find the people and form the group.

One must be careful to implement some basic rules of the group to ensure that the group is not disrupted by any events or persons, and that it remains faithful to the original goal of helping each other to deal with the situations.

15.3 Conclusion

In this chapter we have discussed the method of forming a self-help group of people in similar situations, which can hugely reduce the psychological stress.

Chapter 16: Conclusion

In the previous chapters, we have considered various ways to maintain our mental and physical health and balance the various priorities in life.

We have gone through what is mental health, discussed a few types of mental disorders such as depression, schizophrenia, addiction and stress and discussed some techniques such as CBT and positive psychology to combat stress and improve our well-being. We have also discussed some good online free courses and apps that can positively contribute to our well-being.

It is hoped that application of some of these techniques would help people to handle stressful situations and other responsibilities in a better and more balanced way.

Bibliography

Beck, J. S. (2020). Cognitive behavior therapy: Basics and beyond. Guilford Publications.

Wellman, F. L. (1997). The art of cross examination. Simon and Schuster.

Frankl, V. E. (1985). Man's search for meaning. Simon and Schuster.

Frankl, V. E. (2014). The will to meaning: Foundations and applications of logotherapy. Penguin.

García, H., & Miralles, F. (2017). Ikigai: The Japanese secret to a long and happy life. Penguin.

Hanh, T. N. (2010). Peace is every step: The path of mindfulness in everyday life. Random House.

Hanh, T. N. (2016). The miracle of mindfulness, gift edition: An introduction to the practice of meditation. Beacon Press.

Kabat-Zinn, J. (2013). Full catastrophe living, revised edition: how to cope with stress, pain and illness using mindfulness meditation. Hachette UK.

Skinner, B. F. (1971). Operant conditioning. The encyclopedia of education, 7, 29-33.

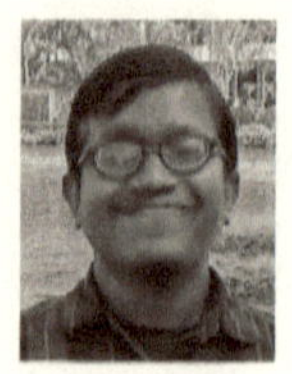

About the Author

Joy Bose is a data scientist and software engineer by profession. He lives and works in Bangalore, India. He has practiced meditation in multiple traditions including mindfulness meditation and Vajrayana, and is keenly interested in applications of technology in the field of meditation.